# Horse 911
*Dr. O'Malley's Veterinary Emergency Handbook*

*Christian O'Malley D.V.M.*

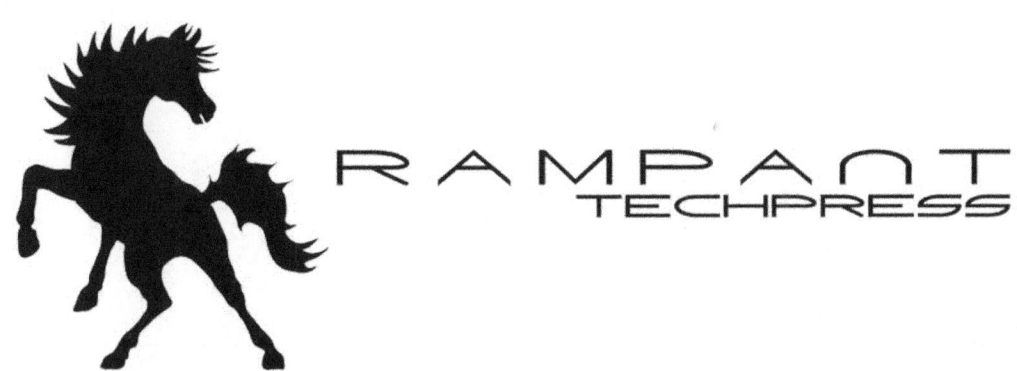

*This book is dedicated to Amy,*

*I Love You.*

*Christian O'Malley, DVM*

# Horse 911
*Dr. O'Malley's Veterinary Emergency Handbook*

By Christian O'Malley D.V.M.

Copyright © 2008 by Rampant TechPress. All rights reserved.

Printed in the United States of America.

Published by Rampant TechPress, Kittrell, North Carolina, USA

Equine In Focus Series: Book #3

Series Editor: Janet Burleson

Editors: Robin Rademacher, Janet Burleson & Teri Wade

Production Editors: Teri Wade & Janet Burleson

Cover Design: Janet Burleson

Printing History:

August 2008 for First Edition

The information provided by the authors of this work is believed to be accurate and reliable, but because of the possibility of human error by our authors and staff, Rampant TechPress cannot guarantee the accuracy or completeness of any information included in this work and is not responsible for any errors, omissions, or inaccurate results obtained from the use of information in this work.

ISBN 0-9759135-3-0

ISBN-13 978-0975913536

Library of Congress Control Number: 2005928013

## *Table of Contents*

Acknowledgement ............................................................................... 1

**Chapter 1: How To Do a Physical Exam** ......................................... 2

  Monitoring a Horse's Vital Signs ...................................................... 2
    *Taking a Horse's Temperature* ........................................................ *2*
    *Respiration* ...................................................................................... *3*
    *Heart Rate* ...................................................................................... *4*
    *The Mucous Membranes* ................................................................ *6*
    *Gut Sounds* ..................................................................................... *9*
  Evaluating the Horse from Head to Toe ........................................ 11
    *The Head and Neck Region* .......................................................... *11*
    *The Body* ...................................................................................... *15*
  What Goes in Must Come Out ....................................................... 21
  Conclusion ...................................................................................... 22

**Chapter 2: Being Prepared for an Emergency** ............................ 24

  What is an Emergency? .................................................................. 24
  Contacting your veterinarian .......................................................... 25
  Making a First Aid Kit .................................................................... 26
  Making a Foaling Kit ...................................................................... 33
  Proper Facilities .............................................................................. 34
    *Fencing* ......................................................................................... *34*
    *Pasture* ......................................................................................... *36*
    *Barn* .............................................................................................. *36*
    *Trailer* .......................................................................................... *37*
  Conclusion ...................................................................................... 38

**Chapter 3: Preventative Care-The Core of Equine Health** ......... 41

  Vaccinations ................................................................................... 41
    *Encephalomyelitis (EEE, WEE, West Nile)* .................................. *41*
    *Encephalomyelitis (VEE)* ............................................................. *42*
    *Equine Influenza* .......................................................................... *42*
    *Rhinopneumonitis* ........................................................................ *43*
    *Strangles (Streptococcus equi)* .................................................... *43*
    *Tetanus (Clostridium tetani)* ........................................................ *44*

*Rabies* ............................................................................................. *44*
*Potomac Horse Fever (Neorickettsia risticii)* ..................................... *45*
*Equine Viral Arteritis* ......................................................................... *45*
*Botulism (Clostridium botulinum)* ...................................................... *45*
*EPM (Equine Protozoal Myelitis)* ....................................................... *46*
*Vaccine Reactions* .............................................................................. *46*
*Intramuscular injection technique* ...................................................... *47*

Deworming ............................................................................................. 52
*Defining a parasite* ............................................................................. *53*
*Other Parasites* .................................................................................. *57*

Anthelmintics ......................................................................................... 57
*Pyrantal pamoate/tartrate (Strongid™)* ............................................. *58*
*Fenbendazole (Panacur™ or Safegard™)* .......................................... *58*
*Ivermectin (Eqvalan™, Zimecterin™, etc.)* ....................................... *59*
*Moxidectin (Quest™)* ......................................................................... *59*
*Praziquantel* ...................................................................................... *59*

To Rotate or Not? .................................................................................. 59
*The Preventicare Program* ................................................................. *60*

The Coggin's Test .................................................................................. 60
Quarantine ............................................................................................. 61
Conclusion ............................................................................................. 61

## Chapter 4: Reproductive Emergencies The Pregnant Mare ............... 63

Normal Gestation .................................................................................. 63
Education .............................................................................................. 64
Breeding Emergencies ........................................................................... 65
Stallions ................................................................................................. 65
*Paraphimosis* ..................................................................................... *65*
*Penile Hematoma* ............................................................................... *67*
*Scrotal hernia* .................................................................................... *67*

Mares ..................................................................................................... 68
*Vaginal Bleeding* ............................................................................... *68*
*Rectal Bleeding* .................................................................................. *68*
*Abortion* ............................................................................................ *69*
*Placentitis* ......................................................................................... *70*
*Dystocia* ............................................................................................. *70*
*Redbag (Placenta Previa)* .................................................................. *79*

Conclusion ............................................................................................... 87
## Chapter 5: Neonatal Emergencies - The Newborn Foal ................... 88
The First 24 Hours ................................................................................. 88
Mare/Foal exam .................................................................................... 92
Environment .......................................................................................... 97
Normal vs. Abnormal ............................................................................ 97
    *Normal Parameters* .......................................................................... 97
Neonatal Problems ................................................................................ 98
    *Prematurity* ....................................................................................... 98
    *Neonatal Maladjustment Syndrome* ................................................ 99
    *Sepsis* ............................................................................................... 101
    *Colic/Diarrhea* ................................................................................ 101
    *Foal pneumonias* ............................................................................ 102
    *Limb Deformities* ........................................................................... 103
    *Umbilical Diseases* ......................................................................... 111
    *Mare Rejection* ............................................................................... 112
    *Neonatal Isoerythrolysis (NI)* ........................................................ 113
Conclusion ............................................................................................ 114

## Chapter 6: Digestive Emergencies ........................................................ 115
Colic ..................................................................................................... 115
    *Colic Examination* .......................................................................... 122
    *What to do when horses colic* ........................................................ 126
    *Causes of Colic* ............................................................................... 128
    *Choke (Esophageal obstruction)* .................................................... 135
    *Diarrhea* .......................................................................................... 140
    *Ulcers* .............................................................................................. 141
Conclusion ............................................................................................ 141

## Chapter 7: Respiratory Emergencies ................................................... 142
Upper Respiratory ................................................................................ 142
    *Airway Obstruction* ........................................................................ 142
    *Tracheal Collapse* ........................................................................... 146
    *Esophageal Choke* .......................................................................... 146
    *Shipping Fever (upper and lower respiratory)* ............................... 147
    *Strangles* ......................................................................................... 147

    *Snake Bite/Blunt trauma to muzzle* ............................................................. *148*

    *Epistaxis* ............................................................................................................. *149*

  Lower Respiratory ................................................................................................ 150

    *Recurrent Airway Obstruction (RAO)/Heaves* ........................................... *151*

    *Pleuropneumonia - Pleuritis and Pleurisy* .................................................... *153*

    *Aspiration Pneumonia* ..................................................................................... *154*

    *Rhodococcus equi Pneumonia (Foal)* .............................................................. *155*

    *Pneumothorax/Chest Trauma* ........................................................................ *155*

    *Synchronous Diaphragmatic Flutter (Thumps)* ........................................... *156*

    *Smoke Inhalation* ............................................................................................... *157*

  Conclusion ............................................................................................................. 157

## Chapter 8: Trauma Emergencies ............................................................... **159**

  Lameness and Injuries ......................................................................................... 159

  Skin .......................................................................................................................... 160

    *Lacerations* ......................................................................................................... *160*

    *Bleeding* .............................................................................................................. *163*

    *Tendon Lacerations* ........................................................................................... *163*

    *Puncture wounds* ............................................................................................... *166*

  Infection ................................................................................................................. 177

  Burns ...................................................................................................................... 178

  Hives ....................................................................................................................... 178

  Acute leg swelling and cellulitis ......................................................................... 179

  Venomous Bites ................................................................................................... 179

  Hematomas ........................................................................................................... 180

  Exuberant granulation tissue (Proud flesh) .................................................... 180

  Foot problems ...................................................................................................... 184

    *Hoof Exam* ......................................................................................................... *184*

    *Emergencies of the foot* ..................................................................................... *188*

    *Hoof Punctures* ................................................................................................. *203*

    *Fracture of the Coffin Bone* ............................................................................. *205*

    *Foot Abscess/Bruise* ......................................................................................... *206*

  Leg Fractures ........................................................................................................ 217

  Conclusion ............................................................................................................. 219

## Chapter 9: Miscellaneous Emergencies .................................................. **220**

  Corneal Ulcers ...................................................................................................... 220

Eyelid lacerations ................................................................. 224
Equine Recurrent Uveitis ....................................................... 227
Seizures ................................................................................. 229
Exertional Rhabdomyolysis (Tying up) ................................. 230
Polysaccharide Storage Myopathy ......................................... 231
Hyperkalemic Periodic Paralysis ........................................... 231
Poisonous plants and Toxins ................................................. 233
Heat stress/ Anhidrosis ......................................................... 234
Allergic reactions .................................................................. 235
Sudden Death ....................................................................... 236
Conclusion ............................................................................ 236

**Index** ........................................................................................ 238

**About the Author** .................................................................... 241

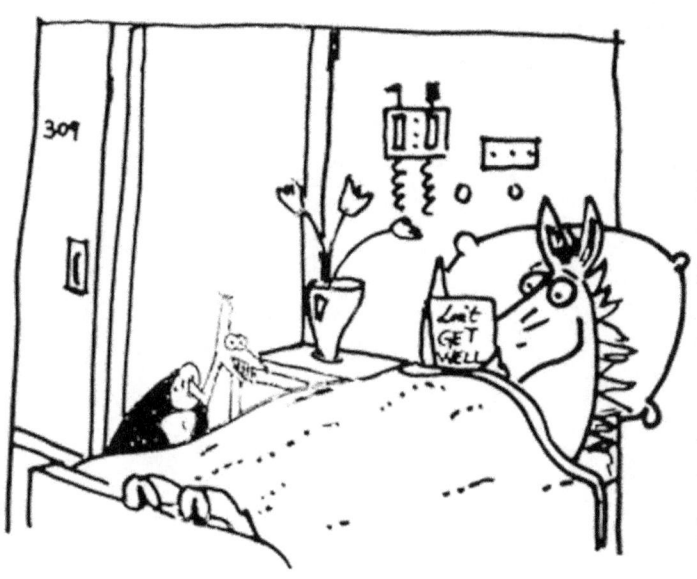

# Introduction

Hopefully this book will be a welcome addition to any horse owner's library. Horse owners are unique in that they are capable of providing much of the care that their injured or sick horse may need. In an emergency situation, this book is a handy tool to reference quickly until the vet can arrive. You may improve your horse's overall outcome potential by following some of the methods described within. Please remember that the advice given here is the author's personal opinion and other methods of treatment may be available.

This book is not meant to replace quality care and treatment by a licensed veterinarian; instead it should be used to complement care provided by an experienced equine veterinary practitioner. I hope that you find the book useful, but will not have to reference it too often!

# Acknowledgement

When Janet and Don Burleson approached me to write this book, I had no idea about the process of preparing a book for publication. Fortunately, they have been there every step of the way with encouragement and insight to get the project done. Many people are involved in the overall production of a book. Without a coordinated effort, the finished work would not be possible. I must also acknowledge my wife Amy, who has helped with proof reading and provided me with the inspiration and assistance to finish the book. There are others such as artists and copyeditors whose names may not be mentioned, but their help with this project has been greatly appreciated.

My sincere thanks,

*Chris O'Malley, DVM*

# How To Do a Physical Exam

CHAPTER 1

This chapter is designed to teach you how to do a physical exam on your horse. Remember, we are not trying to give you a four-year veterinary degree in one chapter, but we are trying to get you to recognize when your horse is normal. So if you know what is normal for your horse, then recognizing the subtle changes in your animal's everyday routine becomes easy.

## Monitoring a Horse's Vital Signs

### Taking a Horse's Temperature

Have your horse properly restrained with a halter and leadline, as well as a handler if one is available. Always stay to the side of the horse when working near the rear of the animal. As you can imagine some horses will react differently to this than others, so be careful not to get kicked. With one arm, hold up the tail and insert the thermometer rectally. Most horses tend to clamp down their tail, so be persistent. Using a digital thermometer is a must for accuracy and speed. Normal for adults is 100 F; foals may range from 99 F to 101.5 F.

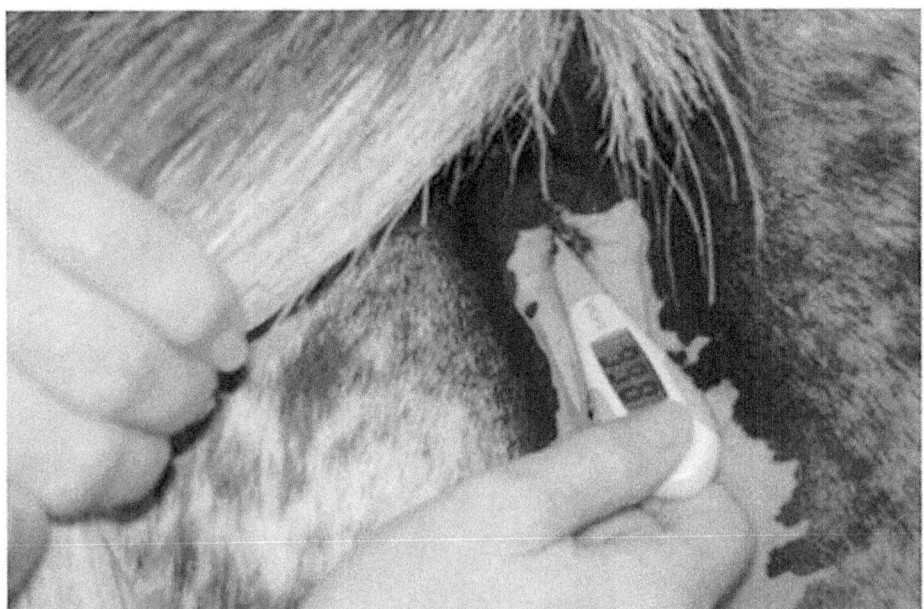

**Figure 1.1:** *Properly Taking a Horse's Temperature*

## Respiration

This is the first section were I will stress how important it is to have a stethoscope. You can not do a proper exam without one. These are available at most drug or medical supply stores for $10-$15. Start by holding the horse in a quiet and stress free environment. Remember your horse's respiratory rate will vary with stressful events and exercise. You may want to practice taking your horse's respiratory rate at different times during the day. Once your animal is in a quiet environment, start by watching his flank go up and down. Count how many times this occurs in one minute. The normal respiratory rate for an adult is 8-12 breaths per minute, for foals it is slightly higher about 20-40 breaths per minute. Another aspect to be aware of is how much effort the horse has to use to breathe. An increased effort can be an early sign of disease. If you really want to do a thorough exam, use your stethoscope to listen to your horse's lung fields. At first, it may be hard to hear anything, but with practice you can start to listen for the normal sounds of your horse's lungs.

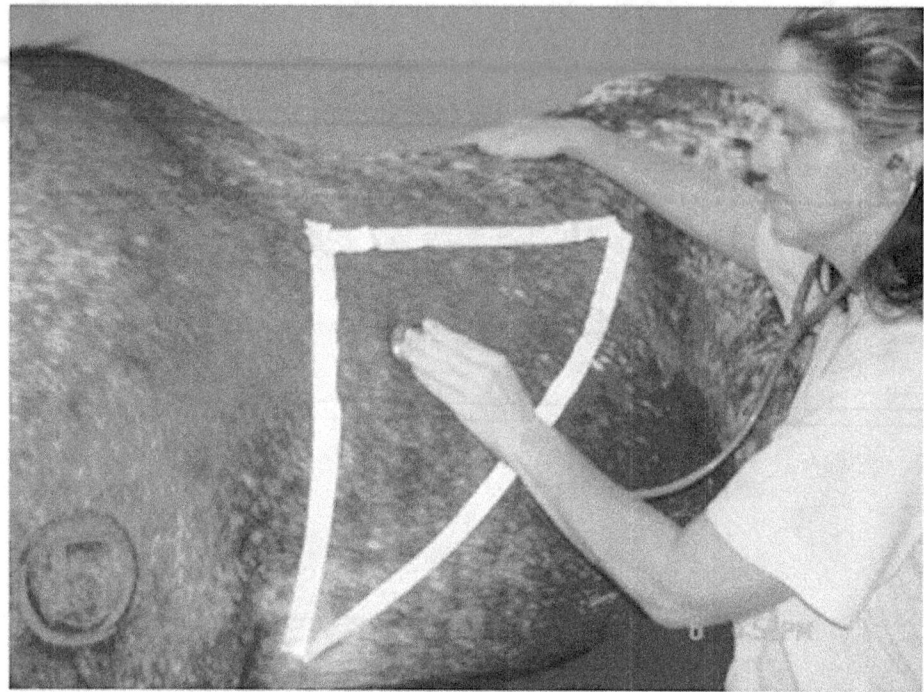

**Figure 1.2:** *Taking a Horse's Respiratory Rate*

## Heart Rate

Once again you will need your stethoscope for this section. The key for being able to hear the heart appropriately is to listen in the right spot. Another couple of helpful hints are to be in a quiet environment and to practice. Remember the old saying "practice makes perfect"; it is true. Always listen on the left side of the horse, the heart is better heard from this side. Place the bell of the stethoscope in the girth area right behind the point of the elbow. Slide the bell of the stethoscope inward between the chest and the elbow a few inches. Make sure the bell is completely touching the skin in that area. Once you begin to hear the rhythmic sounds of the heart, count how many beats you hear in a minute. Remember, lub-dub counts as one beat. The normal heart rate for a resting adult horse is 23-48 beats per minute, for a foal it is slightly higher at 40-80 beats per minute. After you become comfortable, you may be able to tell if your horse's heart is beating normally. Abnormal heart conditions in horses are not common, but can occur occasionally. Being able to pick up on an abnormal beat pattern and rhythm may alert you and your veterinarian of an early problem with your horse's heart. Some horses may miss a heart beat when they are at rest. This condition is called 2nd degree heart block and can be normal in some horses. Try trotting your horse for a couple of minutes then re-check his heart rate. If the problem resolves itself then it is normal for your horse. Make sure you note this in your records for future reference. Heart rate may also be assessed by feeling the pulse inside the lower jawline. The artery here is quite prominent and will move from your finger if pressing too firmly. Try using three fingers. Use your index and ring finger to stabilize the artery and middle finger to feel the pulse. Lastly, the heart beat may actually be seen in the lowest part of the jugular vein just above the chest muscles.

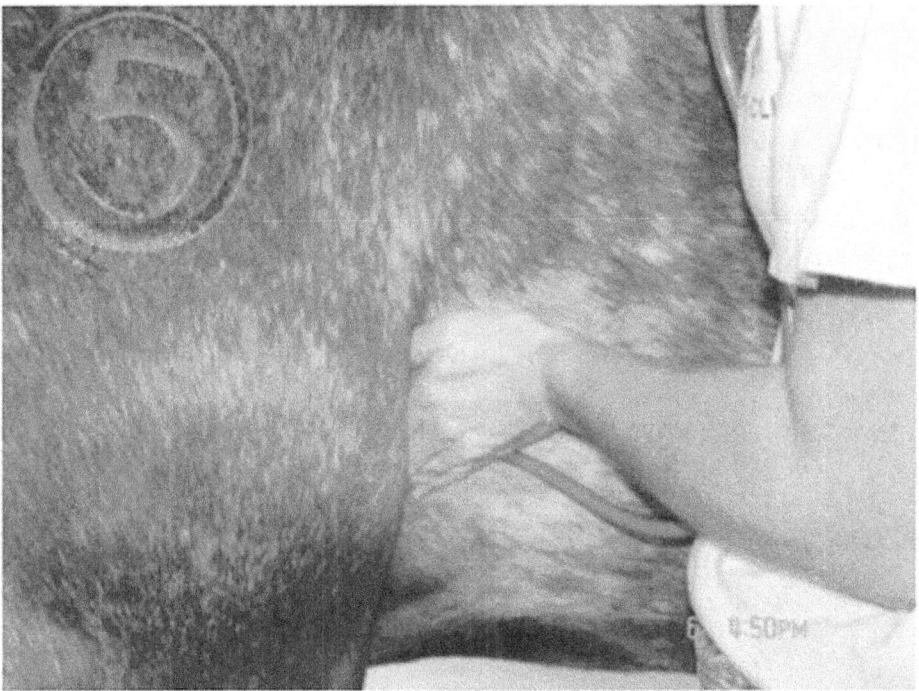

**Figure 1.3:** *Listening to the Heart and Taking the Heart Rate*

## The Mucous Membranes

This to me is one of the most important areas of doing a good physical exam, and probably one of the most informative. Mucous membranes should not be an intimidating term; it is just another fancy way of saying gums. Other mucous membranes can be seen inside the eyelids and inside the vulva. The gums are most commonly assessed. The gum color can range from pale light pink, pink, red, gray, and purple. Each change in color can mean the progression of a disease that all horse owners should consider. The normal color is a light and healthy looking uniform pink. When checking a horse's gums pull up the top lip and check right above the front teeth or incisors. As individual emergencies are covered later in the book you will be provided detailed information about what to do if your horse's gums are an abnormal color, so don't panic!

Another important part of checking the mucous membranes is to also note the capillary refill time. For us regular horse folk, this is a fancy term for noting how your horse's blood pressure and circulation are doing. Do this by pressing your thumb down on the gum above his front teeth and counting how long it takes for it to return to a normal pink color. The magical number is less than two seconds. Anything longer may signify a problem, and will be covered in more detail later, so keep reading.

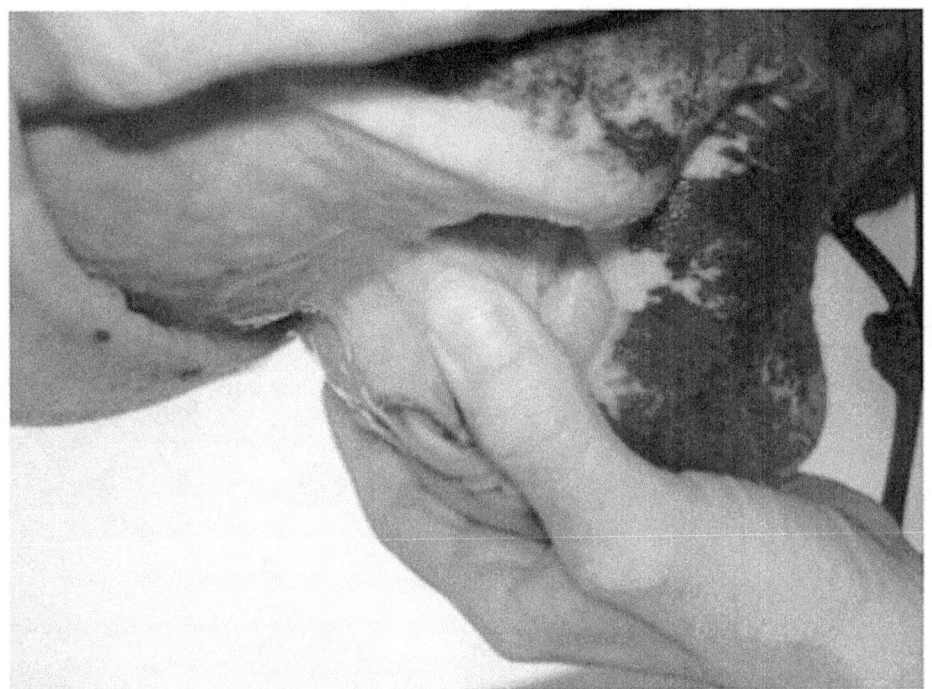

**Figure 1.4a:** *Depressing a Horse's Mucous Membranes*

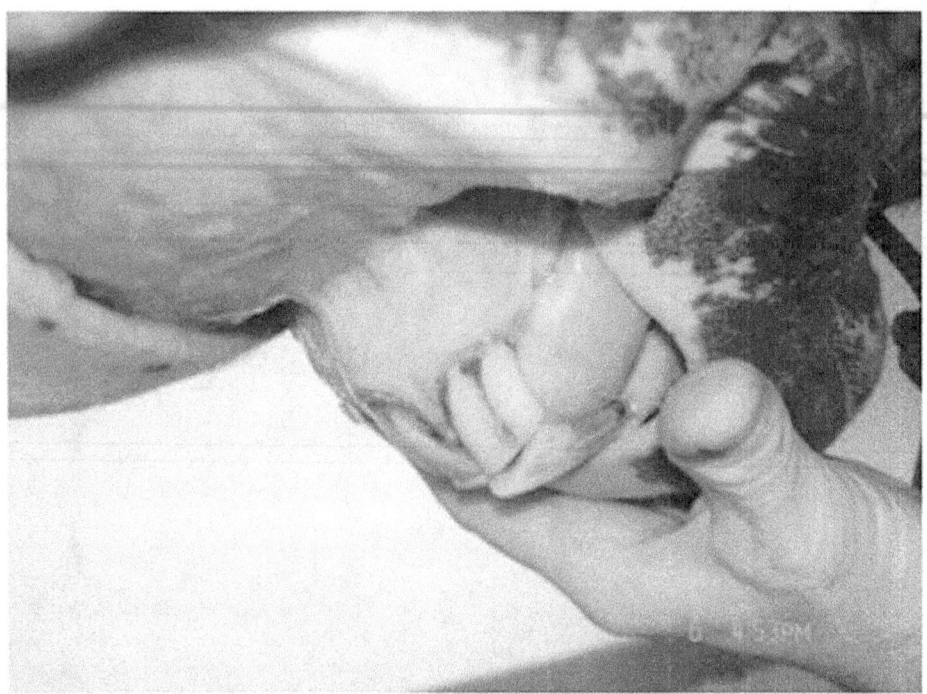

**Figure 1.4b:** *Accessing Capillary Refill Time*

Remember to also note the moistness or absence of moisture in the gums. This can be used along with the skin tent (pinching the skin up and watching it return to normal) to assess hydration. This is best assessed by using the skin in the area of the neck region. From experience I know there are a lot of head shy horses out there, and I have just made checking a horse's gums out to be rather quick, easy and important. Don't give up hope, remember practice makes perfect. Once your horse gets used to you checking them it will hopefully get easier. Also keep in mind, if your horse is not feeling well he will probably let you do anything you want.

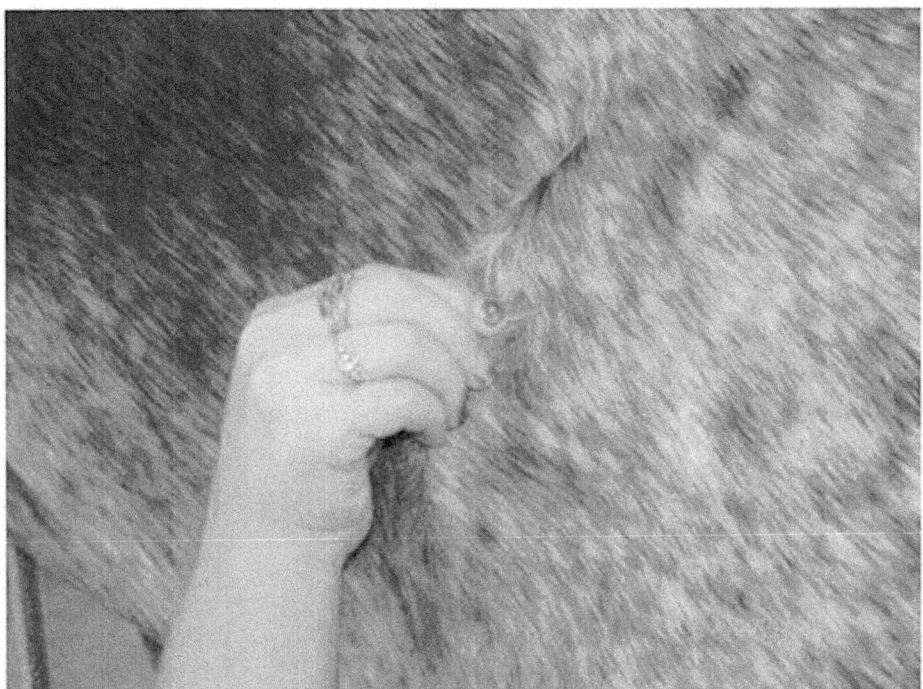

**Figure 1.5:** *Skin Tent for Hydration Assessment*

## Gut Sounds

After the mucous membranes, this is the next part of a physical exam. This is because the majority of emergencies an equine veterinarian treats are intestinal disorders. Or in layman's terms, the dreaded word…colic! Being aware of how your horse's intestines are functioning is an important part of his everyday routine. The keys to being able to hear your horse's gut sounds are where to listen and what to listen for.

There are four easy locations on a horse where you can listen for sounds, and they are as follows. The upper left flank, the lower left flank, the upper right flank and the lower right flank. I have included some pictures at the end of this section to illustrate these areas. Lack of gut sounds in one or more of these areas is a good indication of potential problems in the digestive tract. Some helpful hints when listening are as follows. Once again, make sure you are in a quiet area, then break out your trusty stethoscope and commence listening. Make sure you listen to each quadrant for at least one to two minutes. Sometimes the gut sounds may be just a little depressed. Remember some is a lot better than none!

Now that you know where to listen, exactly what are you listening for? That is a good question, and somewhat hard to explain. I used to own a young horse that would have been a good poster child for gut sounds. You could hear his gut sounds from a mile away! His intestines were constantly gurgling even when he wasn't eating. For the rest of the normal horses in the world use your stethoscope. Gut sounds are similar to what your stomach sounds like at lunchtime in a quiet test hall during a mid-term exam. Even though you are now embarrassed, your horse is proud of his gut sounds, and with good reason. Remember be patient and practice.

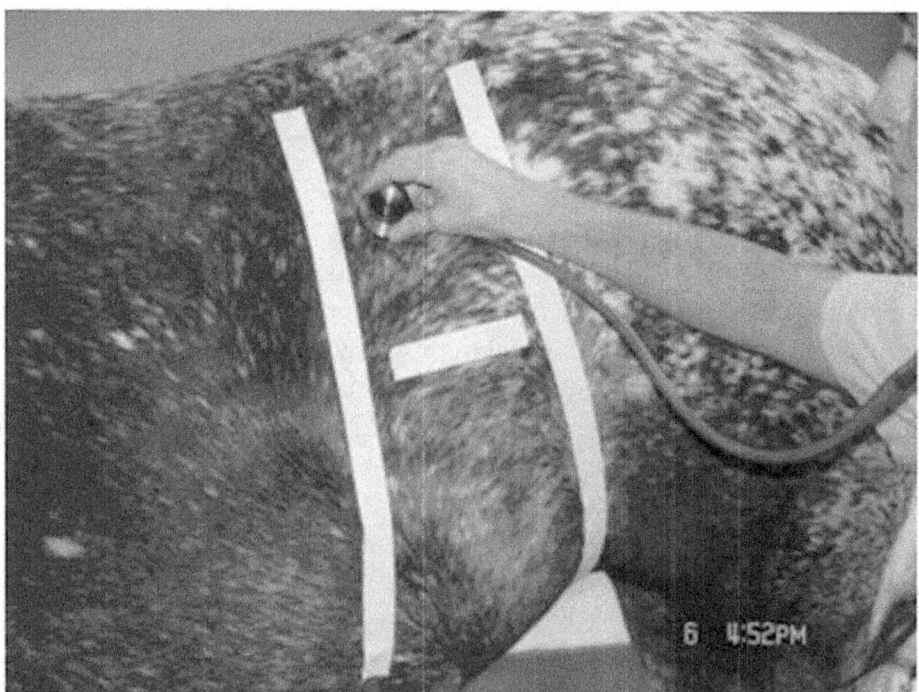

**Figure 1.6:** *The Upper GI Quadrant*

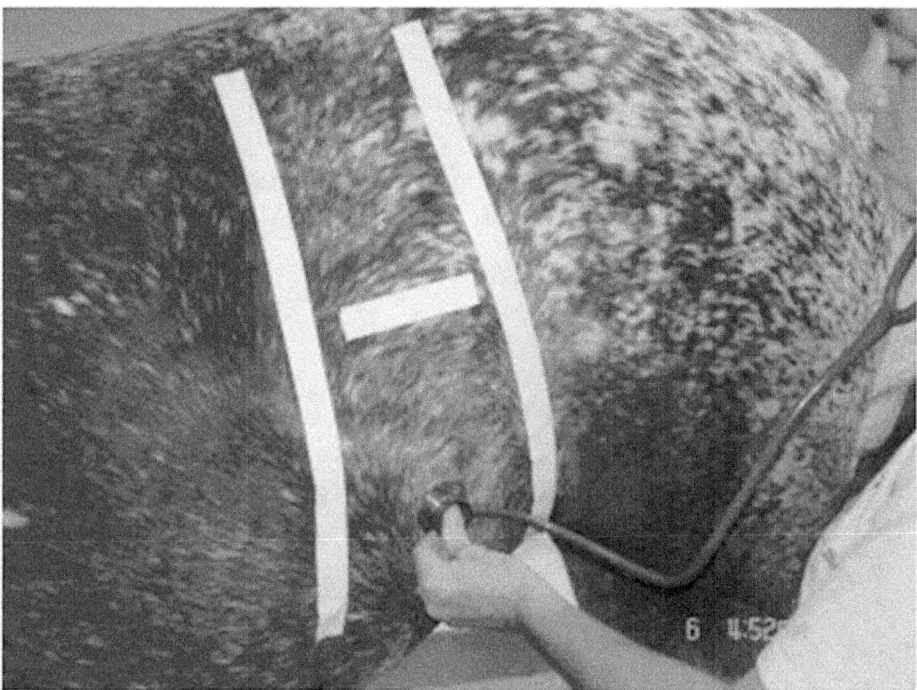

**Figure 1.7:** *The Lower GI Quadrant*

# Evaluating the Horse from Head to Toe

## The Head and Neck Region

Now that we have covered all the important body parameters, it is time to break the body down into different regions and do a brief overview of each. I tend to break the body down into two different sections starting with the head and neck area, and then moving to the body and legs.

First, I start with the eyes. From looking at them with your naked eye to using a good flashlight you can learn a lot. Start by looking at his eyelids, check for any swelling or discharge. Remember a small amount of drainage is normal, large amounts, or any abnormal colors or consistency could be cause for concern. Aside from drainage and obvious swelling, another common sign of trouble is squinting.

Check the surface of the eye for any change in color or for any abrasions or scratches. Keep in mind that it will be covered in more detail later. Eye ulcers need to be evaluated immediately. If you really feel up to a challenge, use a small flashlight to look closer at the eye. Do this in a stall or at least under low light conditions. This can be helpful to detect any problems with the eye's ability to respond to light, and to see if any of the deeper structures are involved.

Many horses are at first shy to the light so never direct the beam perpendicular to the eye. Approach slowly from underneath at a 90 degree angle. Move the light beam on and off the eye until the horse is comfortable with the procedure. FYI: Your horse has a neat little part hanging down from the pupil, and is called the Corpora Nigra or black body. It is believed this helps shade their eye in the bright sunlight and is completely normal. I have included some illustrations on the eye to help. It is so much easier if you can visualize it. Once you become familiar with your horse's eye, you can tell a lot about how he is feeling.

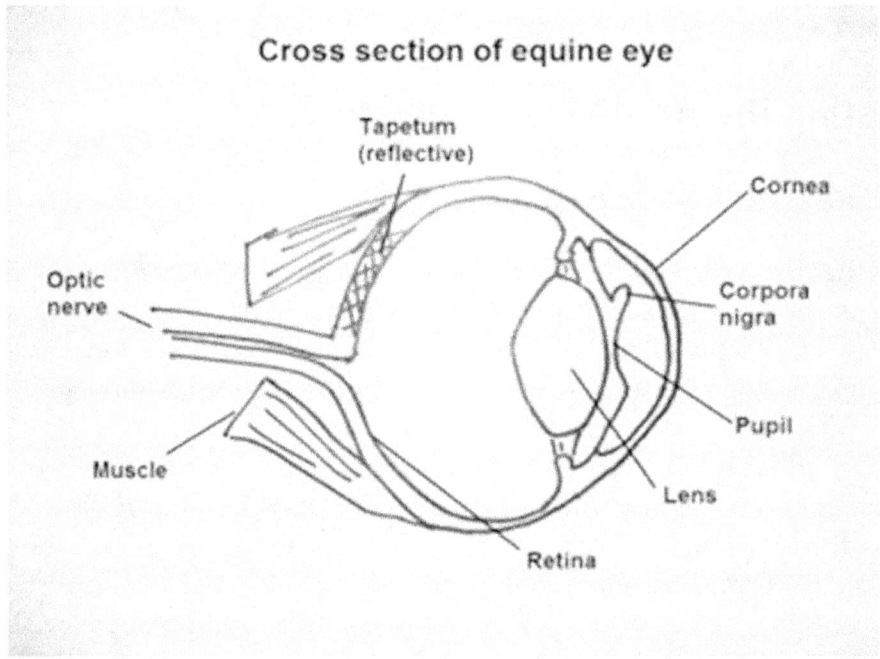

**Figure 1.8:** *Anatomy of the Equine Eye*

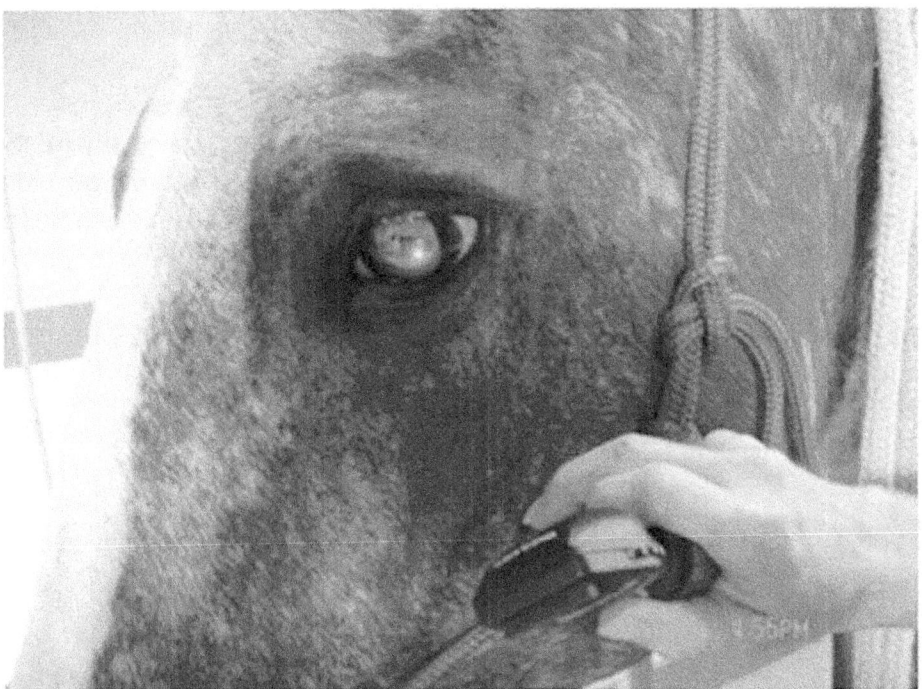

**Figure 1.9:** *Checking the Horse's Eye*

The next area to evaluate on your horse's head is his nostril region. Keep in mind that a small amount of clear discharge seen on occasion is more than likely normal. This can oftentimes be a result of the normal drainage from the nasolacrimal duct, which is the communication between the eye and the nostril region. If on the other hand the discharge is abnormal in color, thickness, or in large amounts you will need to have it evaluated. Another abnormality worth noting is if the drainage only occurs out of one nostril. This is something that may not necessarily be a life-threatening emergency unless frank blood is draining out, but definitely worth discussing with your veterinarian.

Listen to see if your horse has a cough. Just like with a human, a horse with a cold can have both a cough and a nasal discharge. Another item to note is if the animal has a cough, but not any other signs. It is important to investigate the possible causes of the cough and discuss

Evaluating the Horse from Head to Toe

them with your veterinarian. Once again, it is probably not an emergency, but definitely worth discussing.

The last area of the head and neck region to evaluate, especially in young animals is the lymph node region. If they become infected, they can go from the size of a grape to the size of a golf ball quickly. The most common area to evaluate is the slightly depressed area below the lower jaws. Often referred to as the submandibular area, the lymph nodes in this region will become enlarged in the event of local infection or upper respiratory disease. I have included a picture of the submandibular area to prevent any confusion. Now that you have become familiar with the head and neck region, we will move on to the body.

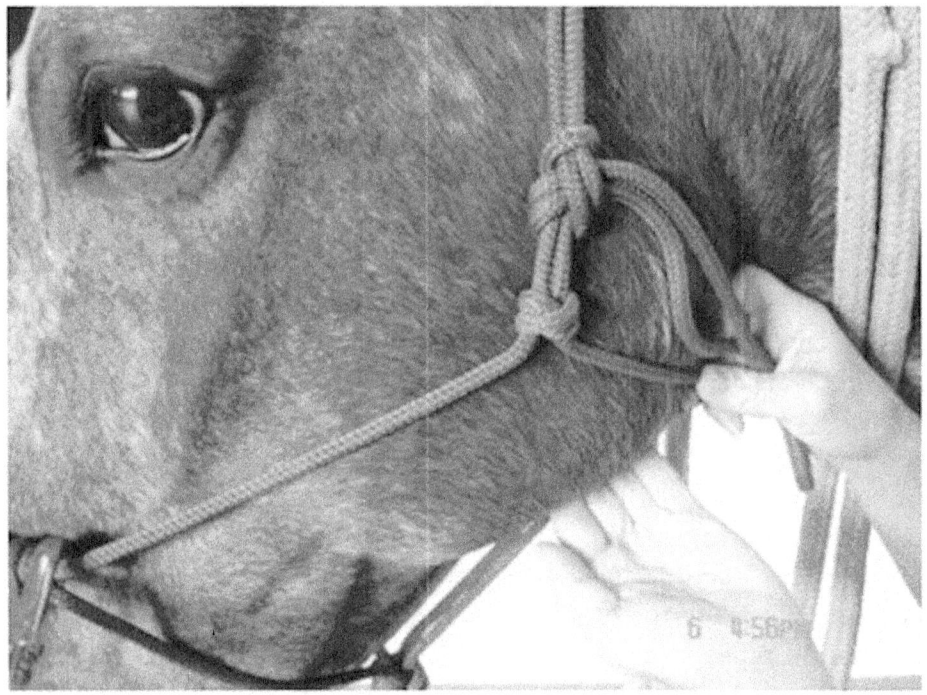

**Figure 1.10:** *Checking Pulse in the Submandibular Area*

## The Body

Once you have evaluated the head and neck region for any obvious signs of concern, it is time to move on to the body. To start, make a quick observation about how your horse is standing, how his body posture appears, and note any obvious cuts/scrapes or masses. How a horse is carrying himself can tell you a lot about where to start concentrating your efforts. For example, if your horse is camped in on his rear-end with his front feet barely weight bearing, do a thorough exam on his front legs. After noting his stance and posture, begin doing your standing exam.

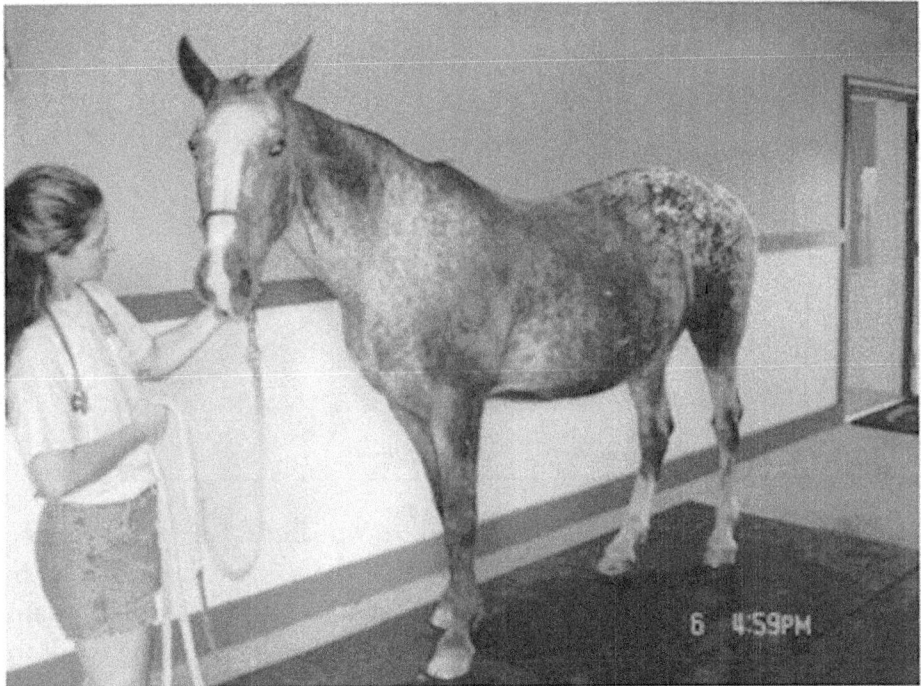

**Figure 1.11:** *Standing exam*

The following image identifies several important point of interest on a horse's body. Use this key when viewing the image: (1) Forelock; (2) Forehead; (3) Bridge of nose; (4) Muzzle; (5) Jaw, cheek or jowl; (6) Throatlatch; (7) Neck; (8) Poll; (9) Crest; (10) Withers; (11) Back; (12)

Loin; (13) Croup; (14) Dock or base of tail; (15) Buttock; (16) Thigh; (17) Gaskin; (18) Stifle; (19) Flank; (20) Point of Hip; (21) Girth; (22) Barrel; (23) Shoulder; (24) Forearm; (25) Elbow; (26) Abdomen; and (27) Chest.

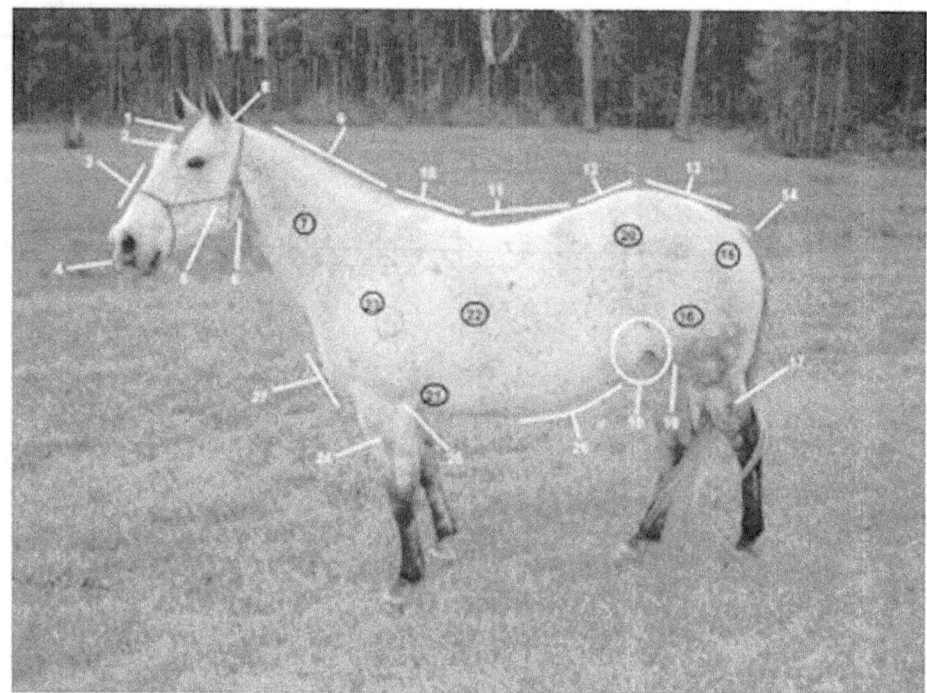

**Figure 1.12:** *Points of interest on a horse's body*

Examine the chest, barrel, flank and rump areas for any swelling or lacerations. After you are comfortable that these areas are normal, begin investigating the legs. It is probably easier to do a thorough exam on each leg before moving on to the next. Start by running your hand down the leg to check for any swelling or cuts. The following figures identify key areas of the leg.

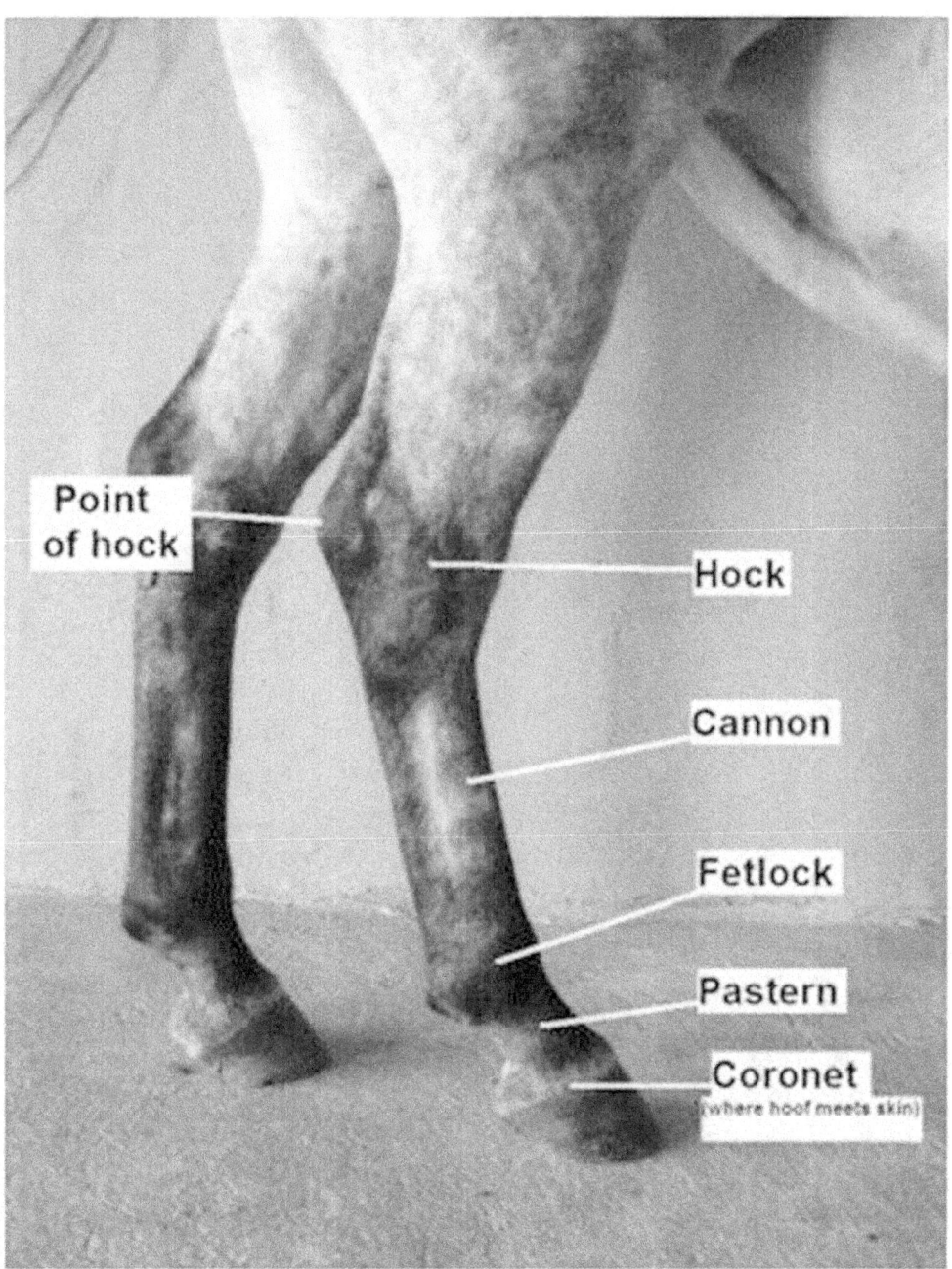

**Figure 1.13a:** *Hind limb anatomy*

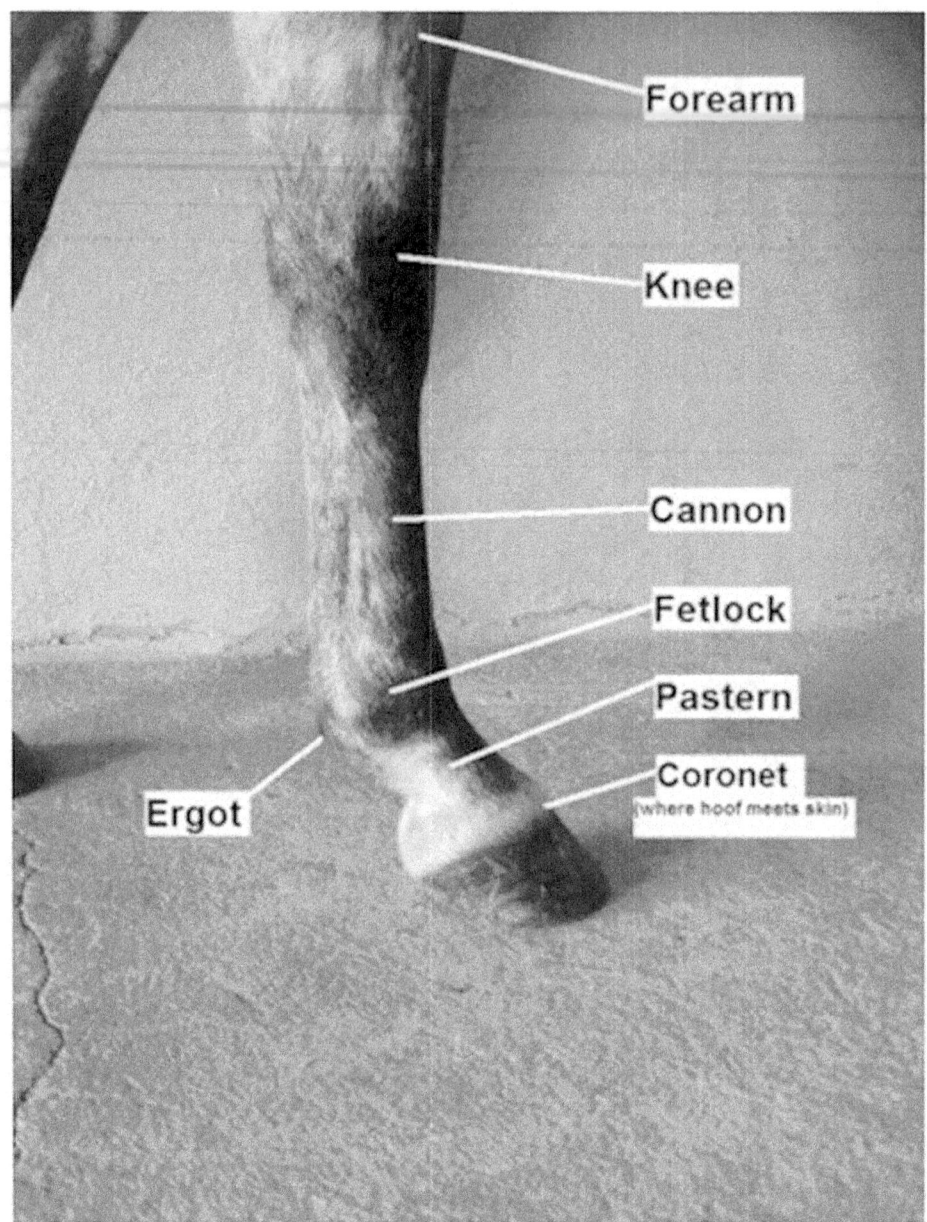

**Figure 1.13b:** *Forelimb anatomy*

Once this step checks out normal, begin evaluating each area of the leg individually. Begin by picking the foot up and checking the underside carefully. Note any odor, abnormal drainage or any foreign objects, such as a nail. Helpful hint, never pull the nail out, let your veterinarian evaluate it first! This will be covered in Chapter 7. Once the foot looks clean, begin manipulating each joint to check for any pain, problems with motion and any abnormal clicking noises. Familiarize yourself with the normal range of motion in each joint. Note any problems with that leg and move on to the next one.

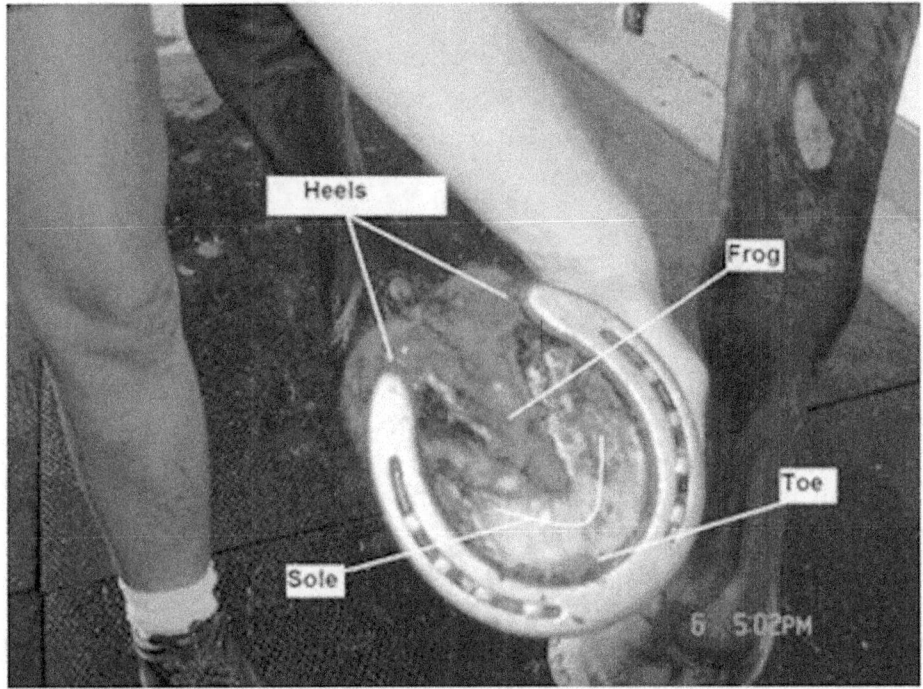

**Figure 1.14:** *Checking a Horses Hoof*

Another item to check on each leg while examining it is the digital pulses. It will take practice to determine where the pulse is and what intensity is normal. I have included pictures that will give a good idea of where to feel for them. Each horse is different, so practice on several different animals.

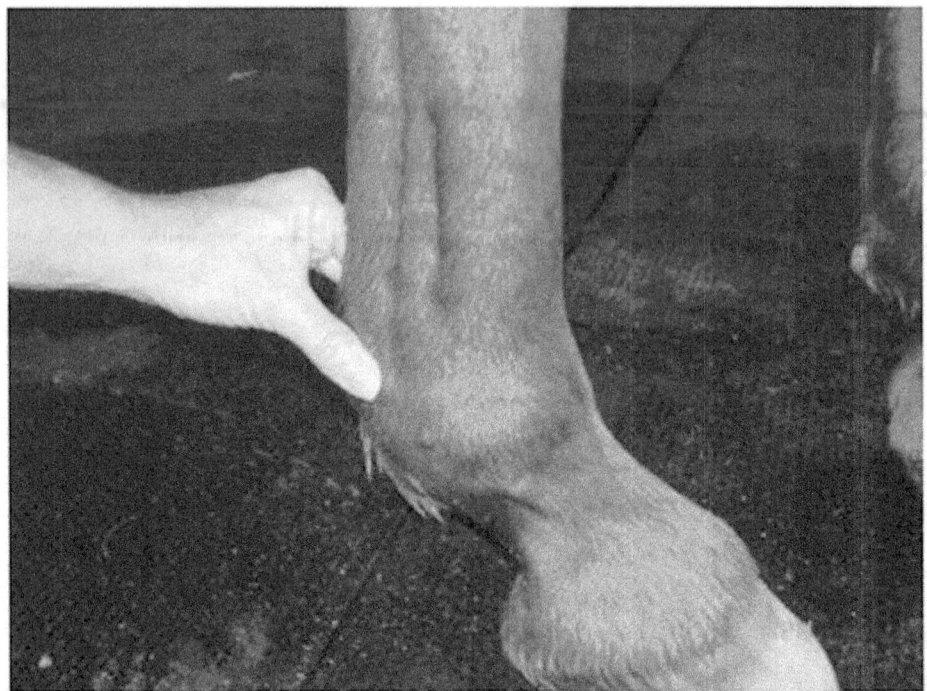

**Figure 1.15:** *Checking a Horses Digital Pulse*

Check all four legs in the same manner and add any changes to your logbook. Remember to evaluate all four legs even if you find a problem with the first one you check, because there may be more than one limb involved. In order to do a thorough physical exam, make sure you check between the front legs, along the belly area, between the back legs and under the tail. Symmetry is an easy way to compare normal from abnormal. So if you aren't sure if a knee or ankle is swollen or enlarged, try comparing to the opposite limb.

Now that you have evaluated your animal from head to toe and are comfortable with your findings, it is time to discuss all of them with your veterinarian. Or is it? What is the first thing they always ask you? Is your horse eating and drinking, followed by has your horse passed any stool today. Since they are going to ask, this chapter will wind up with a short explanation of body functions and their importance in the equine world.

# What Goes in Must Come Out

The most important rule of equine nutrition is to be consistent. Trouble will always come from a rapid change in hay or grain, so choose a good quality feed and stick to them. If you are following these good feeding principles, it will be easy to monitor your horse's food consumption. When an animal does not feel well they will not eat. Be sure to know how much water your horse is drinking. If you are concerned, mark your water bucket and check it every couple of hours. This will be problematic if automatic water dispensers are used or if the horse is kept out at pasture. Bring your horse to the barn and exchange the automatic stuff for an old fashioned bucket.

Now that you are aware of how much your horse is eating and drinking, it is time to cover what is happening on the other end. It is always good to remember that whatever goes in must come out. Once again, if your horse is out to pasture bring him up to a small area so you can monitor him. Any change in color, texture or consistency of your horse's fecal material can be a cause for concern. For instance, a shift to a dark almost black colored stool may indicate digested blood from a bleeding ulcer.

Be aware of any abnormal objects in your horses stool, such as parasites and sand. If you are concerned about sand, set up a quick bucket check. Put some manure collected off grass or shavings in a bucket of water and see if any sand settles to the bottom and note that in your records. But most important of all is if your horse is not passing stool. Any cessation in bowel habits is an immediate cause for concern, so call your veterinarian! Remember that it takes 24 hours for a horse to totally digest and pass what it has eaten through the digestive tract, so a horse can still pass manure and have colic. That is why it is so important to be aware of other signs of colic and not just whether or not your horse is passing manure. All of this will be covered in more detail in Chapter 6 on intestinal disorders. Another item to monitor is urine output. A horse that isn't urinating is a definite cause for concern.

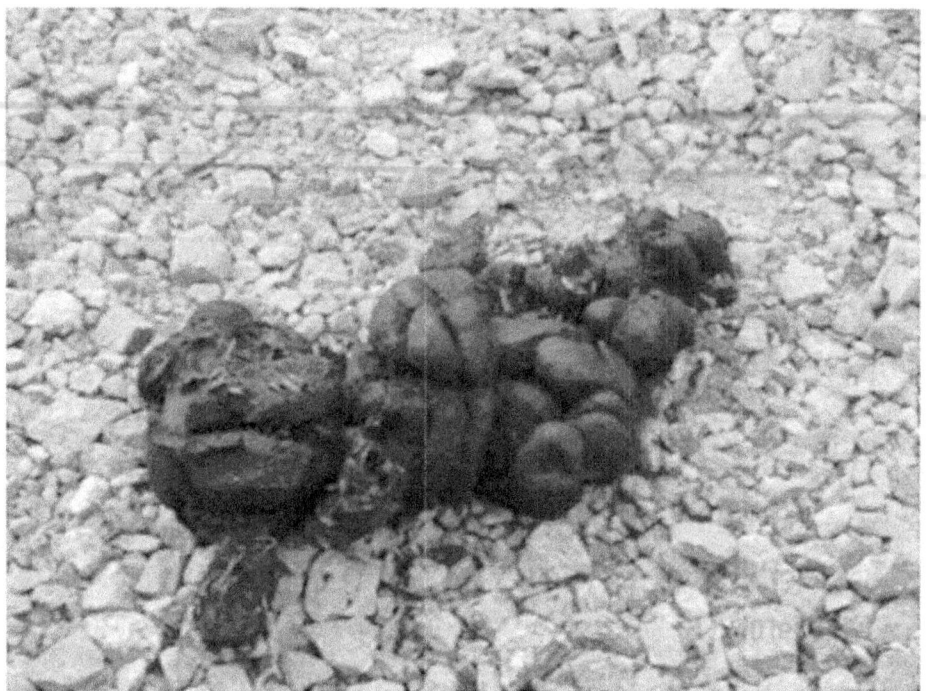

**Figure 1.16:** *Normal Stool*

## Conclusion

The most accurate way to do a physical exam is to do it the same way every time. Once you have a good routine down, you are less likely to forget something. So always start by monitoring your horse's parameters. Once each one has been noted keep track of them in a logbook, so you are aware of any abnormalities. I included a quick reference list to help you remember the big five.

- Temperature
- Respiratory Rate
- Heart Rate
- Mucus Membranes and Capillary Refill Time
- Gut Sounds

After noting all your horse's parameters, next begin evaluating your horse from head to toe. Once again always do your exam in the same way every time so you won't miss anything. Always start with the head and neck region, evaluating the eyes, nostril area and lymph nodes. After you are comfortable with your findings, move on to the body region. Glance over the body and note any abnormalities, then move on to the legs. Remember to evaluate each one individually before moving on to the next one.

After you have done a thorough exam, note if anything is out of the ordinary. Note all changes in eating and drinking habits, even if they are subtle ones. Then move on to noting your horses fecal and urine output.

When all is said and done, you can put all your findings together, and make an educated decision of when to alert your veterinarian. Then together, you can both decide how best to handle your horse and how best to treat his problems. Remember that no one knows your horse better than you!

# Being Prepared for an Emergency

CHAPTER 2

In chapter one, we covered how to perform a thorough physical exam on our horse and to become familiar with what is normal for him on a daily basis. This is what some would refer to as the art of information gathering. Keen powers of observation can alert us to a minor problem before it gets worse. Keep good notes of all the abnormalities you have observed, because when your veterinarian asks, you need to be able to answer them in a quick and concise manner. This will help your veterinarian decide precisely how serious a problem your horse may be having, which brings us to chapter two. This is going to be an informative chapter, because the subjects to follow will help you be prepared in the event an emergency occurs.

## What is an Emergency?

According to Dorland's medical dictionary, an emergency is an unlooked for or sudden occasion, in other words an accident. This book is designed as a teaching tool for horse owners to refer to in the event of an emergency. That way you can confidently recognize an emergency, and know when it is appropriate to call your veterinarian. Most veterinarians do not sit by the phone until the wee hours of the night waiting for an emergency call. The majority of them would rather get a good night sleep instead of going out at three o'clock in the morning in the dead of winter to treat a sick animal. So I am trying to give you all the information you may need to be able to effectively judge a situation and appropriately decide what course of action needs to be taken. If you are dealing with a new problem and not gaining ground on the road to recovery, please alert your vet at the onset, instead of waiting until the weekend or after business hours to get help. Above all, remember that the best way to prepare for an emergency is to prevent one. Each of the following chapters will break down the emergencies most encountered in each body system one by one and explain them in detail. I have included a brief list to follow, so you will know what lies ahead:

- Reproductive(birthing) emergencies
- Neonatal (foal) emergencies
- Digestive (colic!) emergencies
- Trauma (skin/muscle/lameness) emergencies
- Neurologic and Eye emergencies
- Respiratory(breathing) emergencies
- Miscellaneous(poisons, allergies, urinary, genetic, other)

## Contacting your veterinarian

It is a good idea to have a designated area in your barn where you could post all the important numbers associated with your horse. That way anyone taking care of your horses can find them in the event of an emergency.

If you are out of town leave all numbers were you can be reached and a signed authorization for treatment of your animals. We have several clients that call and let us know when they are going out of town and who will be taking care of their animals. That way in the event of an emergency, we can handle it accordingly.

Post all numbers your veterinarian gives you, especially if another veterinarian covers for them on the weekend. If you live in an area that offers more than one veterinarian, try to keep on good terms with both so that you have a backup. After you have concluded that you have an emergency, contact your veterinarian. If the vet does not return your call immediately, try again. Even with all the modern technology available, cell phones and pagers do not always work on the first try. We tell our clients if they do not hear from us in five to ten minutes, try paging us a second time. Leave a clear and concise message always including your name and phone number with area code. After calling your veterinarian, keep your contact number free. It is frustrating for the vet to try and call someone back after they page you only to get a busy signal.

If you receive word that the vet is in route, make sure there is clear passage for them to get to the horse. Move any vehicles out of the way and open gates so they can have their supplies near the horse. Another essential item to discuss with your veterinarian is the location and availability of their facilities. Keep a record on the exact directions to your veterinarian's clinic. You do not want to be driving around for hours looking for their clinic and neither does your horse.

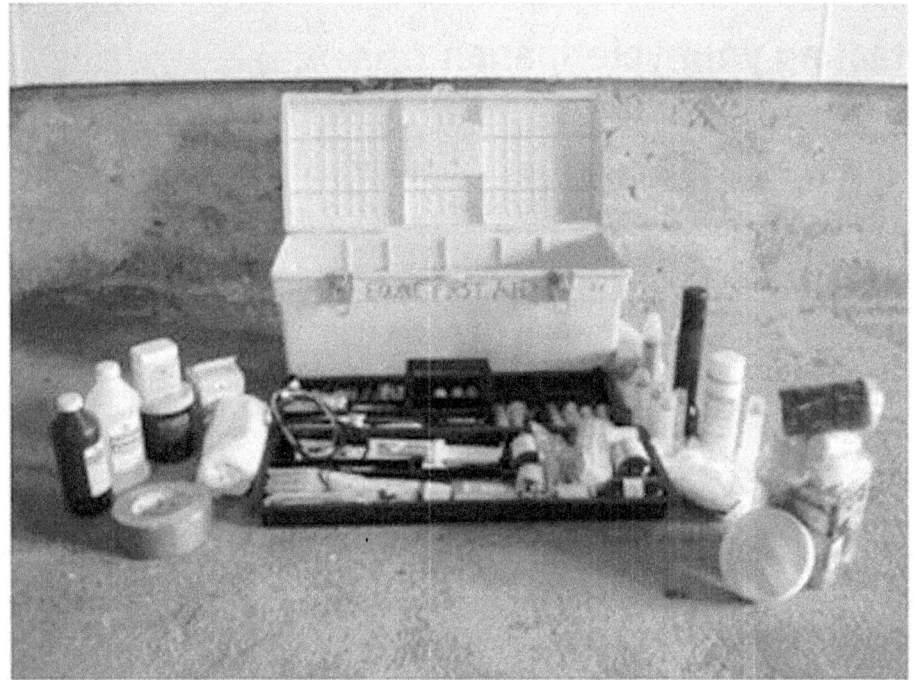

**Figure 2.1:** *Equine First Aid kit*

## Making a First Aid Kit

Your barn is maintained in a safe and proper manner, but nonetheless your horse is not acting normal. Based on your keen observation skills, you make a proper assessment that your horse's condition is in fact an emergency. You have called and discussed the situation with your veterinarian, and they will be there as soon as possible. So that brings us to the next important section of this chapter; what you can have in your first aid kit to help your horse while you wait. Remember that every veterinarian has different ways to treat conditions, so you will want to discuss the contents of your first aid kit with them to see if they have any suggestions. I will give you a list of what I feel is important to have on hand, and then we will review how to properly use each one as we cover each individual emergency.

Another rule of thumb is that the first aid kit should be used for emergencies only. Anything taken out of the kit should be replaced immediately. You do not want to be short of supplies in the event of an emergency. Here is a list and description of First Aid Kit contents:

**Storage container:** You should use a sturdy container with several compartments to organize your supplies neatly. Plastic toolboxes are cheap and great to use. In addition they are readily mobile and easy to grab for storage in the trailer during any transport.

**Flashlight:** Buy a good, sturdy flashlight for your kit. Put new batteries in the flashlight and keep a spare set with it in the container. We use combination LED headlamps. The battery life is much longer and leaves your hands free to work!

**Twitch:** This is an important item to put in your first aid kit because it always seems to disappear when you need it. We prefer the humane twitch. It is held together with some rope at the end and tied to your horse's halter or held by an attendant. When used properly, it will quiet most horses that are being intractable to having a quick or uncomfortable procedure performed. Never rush during the twitching procedure. Take your time, approach the horse slowly, quietly and confidently. Be sure to apply the twitch firmly so that it will not slip off. Some horses can be hard to twitch if they have learned to struggle during the procedure. These horses see the twitch as a painful restraint only and will not have the benefit of experiencing the endorphin release that occurs after the twitch has stayed in place for 3-5 minutes. Try not to leave the twitch applied for longer than 10 minutes. Always have an attendant holding the twitched horse if possible, as some horses can react unexpectedly or "blow up" without any warning.

**Latex gloves:** A box or small bag of gloves can be purchased at your local pharmacy.

**Distilled or bottled water:** It is always a good idea to have fresh water on hand.

**Clean towels:** Our favorites are the blue towels used in hospitals. Regular hand towels will do.

**Syringes:** Keep a large 60cc syringe for flushing wounds or to administer a medication orally. Have a couple of 20cc, 12cc, and 6cc syringes on hand as well.

**Hardware:** Scissors, pliers, a small hammer, and wire cutters. You might have to pull a twisted shoe or cut a tangled fence wire from a leg. Scissors are for bandages and various other tasks.

**Hoof Bandaging Materials:** These are important items to keep on hand especially if your horse has a tendency to have hoof abscesses. It is much cheaper to change your own bandages than it is to have your veterinarian come out every other day for a week and do it for you. Be sure to pay close attention when they are putting on the first bandage so you can see how it is done and know how to change it.

- **Duct tape:** When wrapped properly, duct tape can make a good foot bandage. In the lameness chapter we will show detailed pictures on how to properly make a foot bandage.

- **Epsom salt:** This product has a two-fold purpose. It can be used for soaking the horse's foot when you are trying to draw an abscess out. It can also be used to pack in an abscess once it has been drained.

- **Iodine:** This is also used to pack in the abscess once it has been drained.

- **Cotton:** We usually purchase our cotton by the roll, because it is cheaper. I am not sure if you can buy this at your local pharmacy, so you may want to get a roll or two from your veterinarian. This cotton can also be used to clean wounds.

- **Hoof Boot:** This is a good item to have on hand to put over your duct tape. This helps the bandage last longer and protects a tender sole.

**Regular Bandaging Materials:** These will be the supplies that you use to bandage lacerations and leg wounds. We will show several pictures on proper bandage placement in the chapter on lacerations and their treatment. Some cuts are like hoof abscesses and will have to be bandaged on a regular basis in order for them to heal properly. This will be something you can learn to do yourself, just like bandaging your horse's hoof properly in the event of an abscess.

**Pack of 4x4 gauze:** Gauze is used to put salve directly on a wound and to allow it to stay in close contact with the wound.

**Brown/white roll gauze (3 inch):** This is used to keep the 4x4 gauze snugly adhered to the wound. The key to proper bandage placement is to apply it tight enough to stay but not so tight as to damage the underlying structures.

**Sheet Cotton:** This material is an important part of the bandage. It covers the primary dressing providing extra support. Ask your veterinarian if they carry it or what they recommend in its place. Another popular material is Combi-roll™. Leg quilts are a reusable alternative.

**VetWrap™ (4 inch):** This is the most exciting part of your leg bandage because of the beautiful array of colors to choose from. Whether you choose lime green or black, make sure to use proper technique when putting it on the leg. Remember there is a happy medium between tight enough and too tight. VetWrap is available from your vet and at most feed stores and catalogs.

**Elastikon™ (4-inch):** This is another product you will probably have to acquire from your veterinarian. It is helpful in completing your leg wrap. One roll will go a long way, because all you need is a small amount to wrap around the top of your bandage to keep it from slipping down on the leg. Elastikon™ is similar to the VetWrap™, except with an adhesive backing to help prevent bandage slippage. Scissors are definitely needed to cut it.

**Wound cleaning supplies:** I recommend some plain Ivory™ dish washing liquid to clean off dirt. It would also be a good idea to have some Nolvasan™ (chlorhexidine diacetate) soap to clean the wound itself. You will need to get this from your veterinarian. A bottle of normal saline solutions (0.9% NaCl) is also great. A word of caution: avoid using hydrogen peroxide to clean a wound because it is very tissue irritating.

**Medications:** Every veterinarian has their opinion on owner use of medications so discuss this topic with them first. I will give you my opinion, which is also what I tell my own clients. As I go through them, I will break each one down individually and provide commentary as such.

- **Wound Salve:** This is a special salve that we mix up to use on proud flesh to prevent it from getting worse. We mix it up in our clinic. Basically it helps to promote healing by limiting bacterial infection and abundant granulation tissue (proud flesh). Ask your veterinarian if they have a special concoction of their own that they can recommend.

- **Furacin ointment:** (Wear Gloves) This is good to have on hand to treat small cuts that do not need stitches. I also use this product on mildly irritated skin. Triple antibiotic ointments containing Neomycin, Polymyxin, and Bacitracin serve the purpose as well.

- **Triple Antibiotic Eye ointment:** <u>Prescription only</u>. A safe eye medication to use until the vet can examine. This medication contains **only** Neomycin, Polymyxin, and Bacitracin.

- **Phenylbutazone Paste/Tablets (Bute):** <u>Prescription only</u>. I prefer bute paste over tablets, because it is easier to administer. It is a good idea to keep this medication on hand in the event of an injury. Bute paste works great to alleviate most any pain associated with the musculoskeletal system and to some extent abdominal pain. Bute is often prescribed to help in the treatment of anything from a foot abscess to a swollen joint. Because it is such a versatile and safe product when used properly, Bute is good to have on hand. Before using, discuss the dosage and duration with your vet. Prolonged use or using in young foals can cause gut irritation and kidney problems.

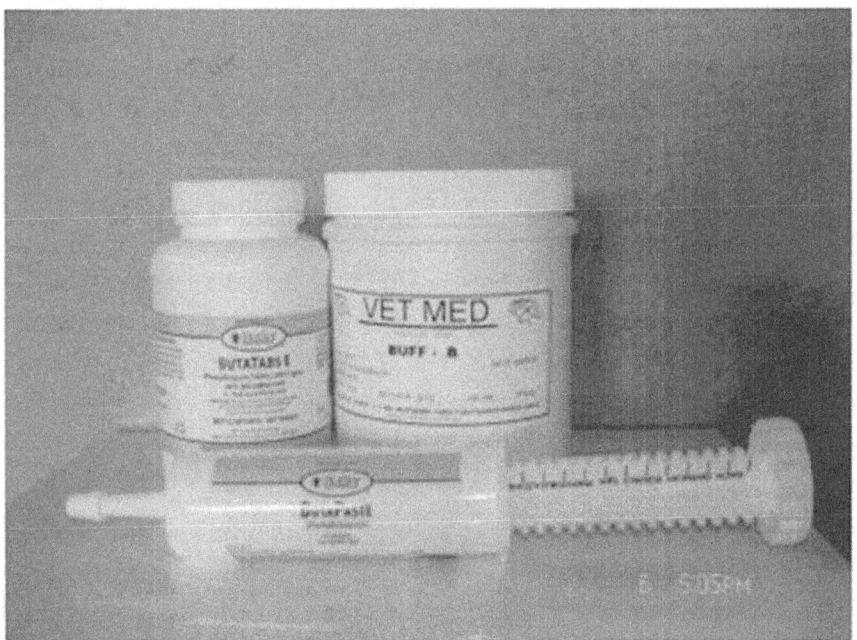

**Figure 2.2:** *Bute Paste*

- **Banamine™** (flunixin meglumine): <u>Prescription only</u>. By far this is the most controversial drug that will be covered. It is also a useful medication for a variety of illnesses. Some people feel that Banamine™ masks the signs of colic and they are right to a certain extent. As with any medication, using too large of a dose can mask certain symptoms. That is why you should discuss with your veterinarian when and how much to use when giving Banamine™. We recommend that some of our clients keep it on hand in case their horse has a mild colic or tying up episode while out of town or in a remote area on a trail ride. The client will call and explain what is going on with their horse and we advise them on what to do if a veterinarian cannot be reached. Once again, I suggest you talk this over with your veterinarian and decide what is right for you and your horse.

As with Bute, Banamine™ can cause stomach ulceration and use should be avoided in foals. This product comes in an injection as well as a paste. Although the injection may be labeled for use intramuscular, we do not recommend going this route. Severe infections and abscesses may develop after intramuscular injection. Use caution! It will probably be personal preference as to which form (if any) you keep in your kit.

- **Antibiotics:** I do not recommend keeping antibiotics on hand, especially if they were used to treat a different problem. Improper use of antibiotics will lead to bacterial resistance. This is an ever increasing problem in today's medical society. Always use antibiotics under the advice of your veterinarian. Penicillin and some other antibiotics are now being sold over the counter at most feed stores and through catalogs. Please do not subject your horse to injections if antibiotics are not needed.

Your emergency kit should go with you wherever your horses go, so store it in your horse trailer when traveling. If your emergency kit contains any prescription drugs, use them only on your own horses and only under the advice of your vet. All prescription drugs should be labeled for the particular patient that is to receive the medication, the amount to be administered, duration of use, and expiration. It is against the law for you to administer these drugs to horses that do not belong to you, even if the owner of the animal consents to the treatment. Simply put, you would be practicing veterinary medicine without a license. Do not take it upon yourself to treat someone else's horse even if you are trying to help. You could end up liable.

# Making a Foaling Kit

These supplies are what I would recommend you have on hand in the event your mare is going to foal. Discuss this and follow the recommendations of your veterinarian as well.

- **Container:** Use a sturdy container to keep all your supplies.
- **Towels:** You will need to have several clean towels on hand. Include some larger towels as well.
- **Trash Bag:** Have a couple of kitchen trash bags on hand to store the afterbirth for later examination.
- **Gloves:** A box of gloves will be useful in case you have to help deliver the foal. Be prepared to save the afterbirth for later examination.
- **Sterile Lubricants:** Water soluble KY jelly is fine.
- **Flashlight:** This has a two fold purpose. One purpose is to check on the mare at night or to watch from a distance without disturbing the mare. Another purpose is to check the baby's eyes after it is born. LED headlamps are great.
- **Enema:** This is to be used in case the baby has trouble passing their meconium, or first stool. Wait until the foal has nursed to avoid any stress or pain with defecation. Fleet™ enemas can be purchased at most pharmacies.
- **Tail wrap:** This is good to have on hand in the event you have to assist in the birthing process. VetWrap can be used since it is easy to use and economical. Remember not to apply the wrap too tight or leave the wrap on too long. Remove it when it is no longer necessary to keep the tail out of the way. Tail wraps are not needed unless you or your vet need to assist delivery.
- **Catch Container:** Have a clean container available to catch your mare's milk in case she is leaking valuable colostrum before the foal nurses.

- **Navel Dip:** There are a couple of different products that can be used to dip the foal's navel. Our recommendation is Nolvasan7 solution diluted one part solution to ten parts water. We think that it works well and has less skin irritation. Iodine is quite irritating on the newborn's skin. It is easy to splash too much on since most foals are quite jumpy during the procedure. That is why we feel it is best to stick to a milder solution that offers the same protection. If the navel is dripping any blood, keep some clean string handy to tie off the cord. There are also sterile disposable plastic clamps that can be used.

## Proper Facilities

The best approach to good horse management is to minimize the risk of accidents. This is best accomplished by keeping your facilities running in a safe and proper manner. This subject will be broken down into different areas in order to provide more detail. The topics include fences, pasture, barn, and trailer.

### Fencing

Make a habit of checking your fence-lines on a regular basis. This includes checking for loose, broken, or splintered boards, nails sticking out, or in the worst case scenario, a down fence. If you find any problems remove your horse immediately and keep him out of the area until the problem is fixed.

The type of fence you choose to put on your farm will dictate the amount of work required to maintain a safe environment for your horse. It is not my place to recommend a certain type of fence, just do your homework and pick the one right for your situation. We will say, do NOT use barbed wire! Remember that fence injuries are quite common for the horse that does not see boundaries in a "scary" situation. Think about durability and visibility when constructing a fence. You may pay more money in the building of a nice fence, but in the long run, less upkeep and fewer injuries associated with the fence will be of financial benefit.

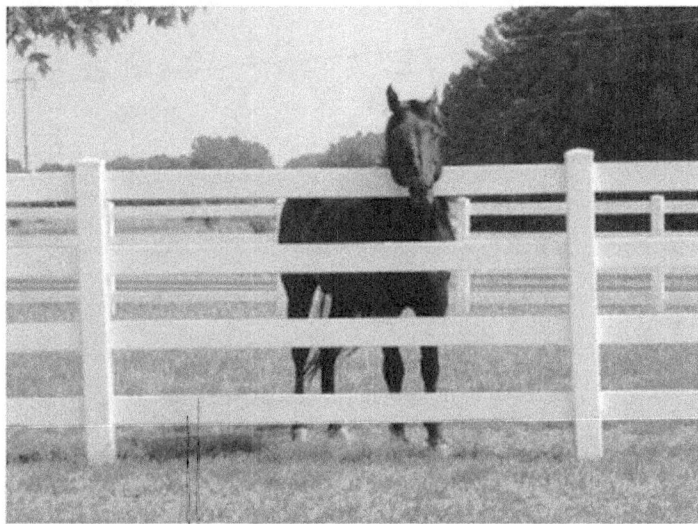

**Figure 2.3:** *Safe fencing*

How to separate horses is another consideration when choosing fencing. Having happy pasture-mates will alleviate injury from fights in the pasture and hopefully from problems across the fence-line. Fences should be at least 4.5 to 5 ft above ground level. Also remember that if you have breeding stallions on your property a good secure fence is a must to keep unwanted pregnancies and fights from occurring. Stallions may need to be fenced inside a 6 ft or higher barrier. Gates should be reliable and easy to open and close. Latches should be "horse-proof" to prevent Houdini-like escapes!

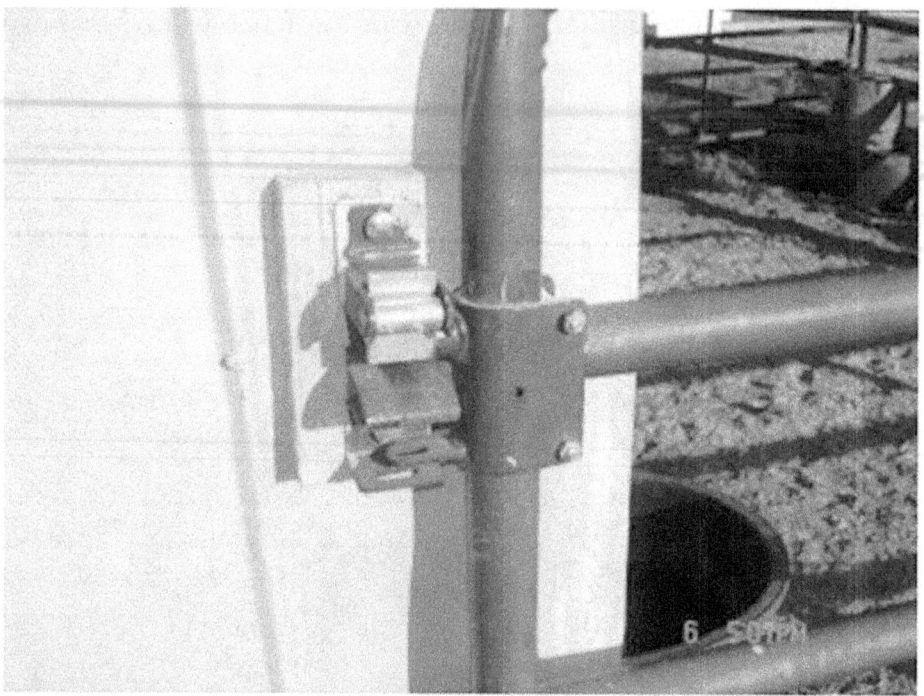

**Figure 2.4:** *Example of a gate latch*

## Pasture

Walk the pasture on occasion to remove hazards. Any holes discovered should be filled. Protruding rocks and foreign objects might surface over time and should be removed when discovered. Familiarize yourself with poisonous plants and trees and get them out of the pasture.

## Barn

No matter how fancy your barn may be, it still must be a safe and comfortable environment for horses as well as the people taking care of them. Having a solid built structure with a proper roof and walls is a must. Install as many fire extinguishers as needed for your size barn. Place signs over the extinguishers for easy identification. Do not allow smoking inside the barn. Almost everything in a barn is combustible! Install smoke detectors where applicable.

Monitor each individual stall much like you do your fences. Look for any loose boards or nails sticking out. No matter what type of stall door you have remember to keep all stall latches in their proper place and the doors wide open when moving horses in and out. Also keep the aisleways free of debris so horses can move in and out in a safe manner. The footing will depend on the type of barn you have, but maintain it in a safe and proper manner for your individual circumstance.

Another key item is to always keep all the doors locked and escape proof. This is of paramount importance when dealing with the feed room. Many a horse has had to be treated for grain overload after successfully letting themselves into the feed room and eating to their heart's content. Having a sheltered work area with proper lighting and access to water is important in the event of an emergency. Without these amenities your veterinarian could be limited in what they can do for your horse. If you do not have these facilities available, have a plan in mind so you can provide them. Now we can turn our attention to the trailer.

## Trailer

This brings us to another important topic. It is important to have access to a trailer. Every horse owner should have a trailer or at least have access to one. This may mean borrowing a friend's or using a commercial service, either way, have a plan in mind in case one is needed.

Another necessity is to make sure your trailer is working properly. Nobody wants to get half way into a trip to the veterinary clinic at two o'clock in the morning and break down on the side of the road. We keep a locked toolbox affixed to our trailers that contain extra ropes, tire changing equipment, pliers, and a hammer. If your trailer breaks down in route to the hospital, having the necessary equipment and spare parts is easier than waiting for a second trailer to arrive. Keep in mind there are few emergencies that would prohibit a trailer ride to the clinic. This actually may be the best option for your horse, because in the long run being in a hospital setting may be ideal. In some cases, you or your vet may need to stabilize the horse prior to travel with bandaging, splints, or pain medications.

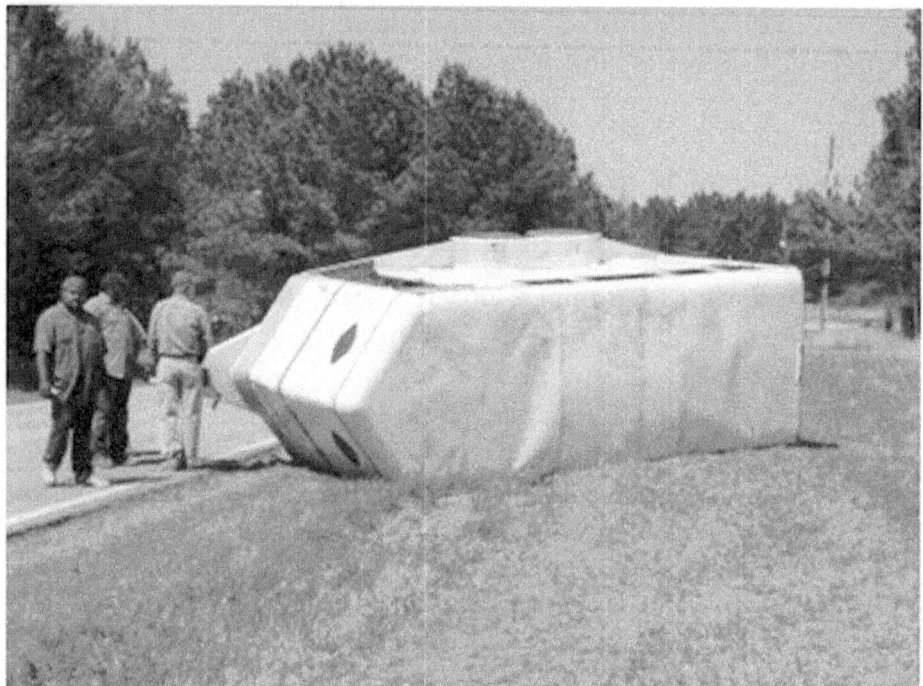

**Figure 2.5:** *Detached trailer – Use correct size ball and chains!*

Now that we have our fences, facilities, and trailer ready, it is time to move on to the next section, which is the core of equine health.

## Conclusion

As a keen observer we know how to decide when we need to contact the veterinarian to discuss the possibility of an emergency. Then in the chapters to come we will explore what we can do for each emergency while we wait for the veterinarian to arrive. Since this chapter was full of important material, I thought it would be good to sum up some of the ideas.

## Contacting the Veterinarian

- Post all important contact numbers for your veterinarian in central location in the barn
- Leave clear and concise message, remembering to leave name and number
- Keep contact number free so your veterinarian can get in touch with you
- Move vehicles and open gates so the vet can get close to the horse

So your veterinarian is on their way, what can you do while you wait? That will depend on what you have in your first aid kit.

## The First Aid Kit

- Keep all your supplies in a good container
- Replace all used items immediately
- List of items-flashlight, gloves, clean towels, distilled water, twitch, hoof bandaging materials, regular bandage materials, wound cleaner, and medications
- Discuss all supplies with your veterinarian-where to locate, how to use and anything else they suggest

We have successfully assembled our first aid kit, so now it is time to put together a foaling kit for our pregnant mare.

## The Foaling Kit

- List of items-container, gloves, towels, enema, tail wrap, catch container and navel dip
- Recommend Nolvasan7 solution as the navel dip because it is less irritating

This brings us to our final concluding summary of this chapter, which is how to maintain our facilities in proper order.

**Facilities**

- Check barns, fences and pasture on a regular basis for potential hazards
- Have access to good working environment-dry area, lights, and access to water
- Have access to properly working trailer-friends, or commercial service

So now that all the important take home ideas are organized in a few lists, this brings us to the end of chapter two. Above all, I hope this book is giving you some resourceful information you can use in the event an emergency occurs. Now before we break down each individual disease process, we will take a step back and concentrate on the core of equine health, which is preventative care.

# Preventative Care-The Core of Equine Health

CHAPTER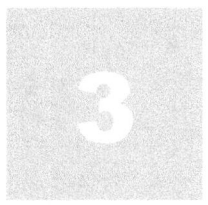

This brings us to another important chapter on how to keep your horse healthy. Instead of covering this in chapter 2, we decided to give this topic more attention since it is the core of equine health. The subjects are as follows: vaccination, de-worming, quarantine, and the Coggins test. We will cover each topic in detail, and give you helpful guidelines. As with the previous chapters, I have stressed how imperative it is to discuss these ideas with your veterinarian and individualize them for your own horse's health program.

## Vaccinations

A vaccination is when an animal is given an antigen for a specific disease in order to stimulate the animal's immune system to actively fight off that disease if challenged with it in the future. Be aware that no vaccine can prevent a given disease 100%. If the animal is properly vaccinated and still contracts the disease, it is often not as severely debilitated and can, in most cases, recover.

There are many vaccine companies out there and it is not my place to recommend one over the other. I will just give you the most appropriate way to use each vaccine. Although most vaccines come in several different combinations, I will break each one down individually. Lastly, the types of vaccines your horse will need depend on variables such as age and type of use.

### Encephalomyelitis (EEE, WEE, West Nile)

This includes:
- Eastern Equine Encephalitis (EEE)

- Western Equine Encephalitis (WEE)
- West Nile Viral Encephalitis (West Nile)

These diseases are spread by mosquitoes. Birds, horses, and humans can contract the diseases by being bitten by a mosquito harboring the virus. Depending on where you live in the country will dictate how often you will need to vaccinate. In the southeast, where the mosquito season can be year-round, we recommend vaccinating twice a year--in the Spring and Fall. The first dose needs to given when a foal is 3-4 months of age, and then repeated 3-4 weeks thereafter. Broodmares should be vaccinated 30-45 days before foaling. There will be more on broodmare vaccination in the next chapter.

In North Carolina, the state veterinarian monitors confirmed cases of encephalitis and will make recommendations for any change in vaccination protocols. During various times it has been recommended to vaccinate 3-4 times a year. This is a decision about which you may want to confer with your veterinarian first, but twice a year is ideal. Following vaccination protocol is a must to help keep your horse healthy and free of disease. In addition to vaccination, you can take measures to remove standing or stagnant water in your environment to limit the breeding grounds for mosquitoes.

## Encephalomyelitis (VEE)

This section will cover Venezuelan encephalitis, which usually only comes in combination with eastern and western encephalitis. This vaccine is usually only given in endemic areas or in the threat of an outbreak. If needed, it should be given once a year, on a Spring rotation. If necessary, as with EEE/WEE, Fall boosters may be indicated in endemic areas. As above, the first dose is given at 3-4 months of age and then again 3-4 weeks later.

## Equine Influenza

The influenza vaccine is one that I will break down by discipline and age because this will dictate how often you will need to vaccinate. The viral disease is spread between horses by direct contact, aerosolization, or indirectly via contaminated objects (clothing, tack, etc). For young or performance horses, it is recommended that you vaccinate every three months. On the other hand, brood mares and pleasure horses will only need the vaccine twice a year. It is advised that you booster mares 30-45 days prior to foaling. In foals, the first dose is give at 3-6 months of age, followed by two booster shots at one month intervals.

## Rhinopneumonitis

Referred to commonly as Equine Herpes Virus - Type 1 (EHV1) and type 4 (EHV4). This vaccine is often presented in combination with the above vaccines and is dosed in a similar fashion. EHV1 is a virus spread between horses by direct or indirect contact. The virus can cause respiratory, neurological or reproductive (abortion) problems. EHV4 primarily causes respiratory problems. The timing for giving the rhinopneumonitis vaccine (EHV1/4) is dictated by age and discipline. For young and performance horses, it is recommended every three months. For pleasure horses the vaccine is done twice a year or not at all. For the majority of our older, retired, or backyard horses, we do not usually vaccinate for this disease. It is recommended that broodmares receive the EHV1 component of the vaccine at the 3rd, 5th, 7th, and 9th month of pregnancy to prevent abortions associated with this virus.

This particular vaccine, often referred to as the Pneumabort-K™ vaccine, is not the same what is used in the pleasure and performance horses, which contains both EHV1 and EHV4. Broodmares should receive the EHV1/EHV4 vaccine before breeding and again 30-45 days before foaling.

## Strangles (Streptococcus equi)

The Strangles vaccine is can be important for young horses where the disease can spread rapidly. It is caused by bacteria and is highly contagious from horse to horse by direct or indirect contact. Excretions from an infected horse contain abundant bacteria which can live in the environment for months. This disease usually occurs in outbreaks in larger breeding barns or places where many horses frequent such as sale arenas, show grounds, quarantine facilities and from time to time larger boarding/training barns. Here again, the use of a strangles vaccine depends on the environment or type of travel your horse is exposed to.

Annual vaccination in the Spring is our recommendation. Bi-annual vaccination can be performed in areas of high risk. If an outbreak occurs, vaccination of horses in the nearby vicinity may be warranted. The first dose is usually given around 6 months of age with a booster a month later. There are different vaccines available, but we always use the intranasal preparation because it has fewer side effects.

## Tetanus (Clostridium tetani)

We recommend this vaccine once a year and it is often presented in conjunction with several of the above vaccinates. It is necessary to booster this vaccine in the event of injury or surgery. The first dose is given to foals at 3-4 months of age and then again a month later. Broodmares should be vaccinated 30-45 days before foaling.

## Rabies

This disease is endemic in several areas of the country and should be recommended accordingly. Rabies is a viral disease spread between all mammals directly from the saliva of the infected animal. This can occur either from a bite or merely having the saliva contact broken skin. Symptoms will be discussed in the neurological chapter. In the southeast we advise our clients to give the rabies vaccine once a year. This vaccine is relatively inexpensive and is a must due to a certain death sentence for animals that contract the virus. In addition, there is a public health concern since humans can potentially contract rabies from any infected animal. For foals the first dose is given at 3-6 months of age and boosted a month later. Broodmares are vaccinated 30-45 days before foaling.

## Potomac Horse Fever (Neorickettsia risticii)

Potomac Horse Fever is generally recommended in endemic areas only. This is usually any state in the Potomac River region or one that has had outbreaks of the disease in the past. Although the transmission of this disease is not 100% certain, there is an intermediate host, possibly a snail, needed to complete the lifecycle. Symptoms include a high fever and profuse, watery diarrhea.

Keep in mind that if your horse is traveling into one of the states in this region for any reason, you may want to vaccinate them. For all ages and disciplines the vaccine is recommended on a yearly basis. The first dose is administered at 3-4 months of age with a one month booster.

## Equine Viral Arteritis

This vaccine is only used with extenuating circumstances and its use depends highly on state regulations. It is mainly used in breeding animals. Mares should be vaccinated at least three weeks prior to being bred to a positive stallion. However, they should not be vaccinated in the last two months of pregnancy. Stallions on the other hand can be vaccinated at least three weeks before breeding season. Keep in mind that vaccinated animals may not be able to be exported to other countries because of seroconversion. This is the presence of the antibody in blood after vaccination. Use it only when necessary.

## Botulism (Clostridium botulinum)

Only give to animals in endemic areas or ones that travel to such areas. It is an annual vaccine and for broodmares can be given 4 weeks prior to foaling. The initial three dose series is given at 30 day intervals and is started at the age dictated by what is appropriate for that area.

## EPM (Equine Protozoal Myelitis)

EPM is a protozoal disease affecting horses nationwide. The disease can cause various neurological signs in any age horse. The disease can be endemic in certain areas or only affect a single horse on a farm. Most horses that are exposed to the protozoa do not develop symptomatic disease, however roughly 60% or more will show a positive result for the antibody in the blood. This means that the horse has been exposed in their lifetime with or without showing symptoms. A vaccine was developed and approved for use in horses in the early 2000's. In the early stages of the vaccine's release, there was skepticism as to whether immunity or even partial immunity could be achieved since EPM is a protozoan rather than viral or bacterial disease. Also, some veterinarians are concerned that vaccinated horses will show a positive result for EPM antibody in their spinal fluid thereby making interpretation of this diagnostic test obscure. Your veterinarian can instruct you as to what is appropriate for your horse and your area.

## Vaccine Reactions

In most cases, vaccinations are given without any subsequent reaction. However, there is a risk for vaccine reaction to occur. The reactions are usually local swelling and/or stiffness in the area where the vaccine was administered. In a few cases, a severe anaphylactic reaction might occur which could lead to death.

Anaphylaxis will typically have a sudden onset within minutes. Some of the signs may include increased and shallow respiration, anxiety, hives, and sweating. Treatment with IV epinephrine is preferred to help quell the body's adverse reaction. If you feel that your horse is having an anaphylactic reaction, contact you veterinarian immediately.

Local vaccine reactions such as swelling and pain are, as mentioned earlier, more common and easier to manage. Keep these horses moving and discuss with your vet whether to administer an anti-inflammatory. If several horses have reacted to a particular vaccine, there may be a problem with the vaccine itself. Do not use the remaining portion and contact the vaccine manufacturer. Here are a couple pointers to help decrease the chance of a vaccine reaction:

- **Use clean needles!** This sounds like a no-brainer, but here is my idea of a clean needle: If you pull up the vaccine from a multiple dose vaccine bottle, do not use the same needle to inject the horse that was used to stick the bottle. Also, if you inject the horse and for some reason the horse moves away before completing the injection, do not re-insert the same needle. Use another. It will be worth the extra ten cents to avoid a reaction. Wipe the top of the vaccine bottle with an alcohol wipe before pulling up the vaccine.

- **Inject clean horses!** Another no-brainer. Avoid mud-caked areas, sweaty, and wet areas. If necessary, curry comb a small area, wipe the injection site with alcohol, and wait for the area to dry.

- **Store vaccines properly, and in a refrigerator.** Watch for expiration dates and do not use expired product. Many vaccines have a pH color indicator that lets you know if something has changed in the vaccine or becomes contaminated. Also, do not mix different vaccines in the same syringe. This may decreases the efficacy of the product.

## Intramuscular injection technique

Knowing how and where to give intramuscular injections is important if you own or care for horses. Many medications including anti-inflammatory medications, antibiotics, vitamins, and vaccines can be administered via injection. Be sure that the medication is designed to be given in the muscle and always use sterile needles and syringes. After needle insertion, pull back on the syringe plunger to ensure the needle has not inadvertently entered a vessel. If blood flashes back, simply redirect the needle to another area. After injection, briefly massage the area to disperse the medication.

## Neck

The neck is a very common site for intramuscular (IM) injection. The benefit of using the neck is its safety for the handler as well as a better area to treat should a reaction or infection occur that is secondary to injection. If standing on the left side if the horse, place your right hand palm down on the neck, keeping your fingers pointed towards the ears. Slide your hand down the middle of the neck until the heel of your hand reaches the shoulder. At this point, your preferred injection site would be between your knuckles and finger tips. This falls about 4-6 inches in front of the line formed from the shoulder to the withers. The injection area forms a triangle.

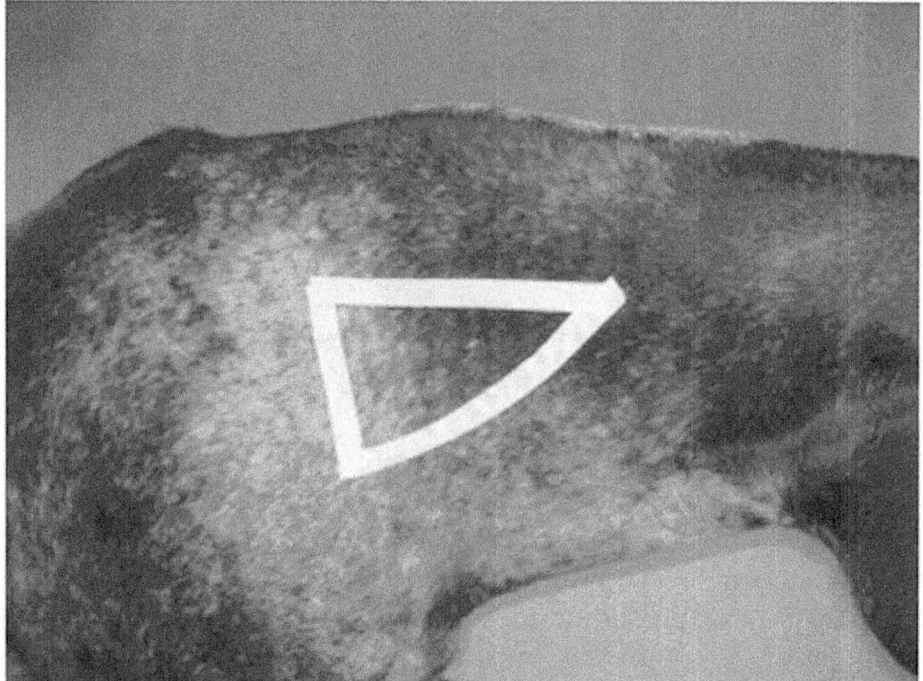

**Figure 3.1a:** *Intramuscular injection site on the neck*

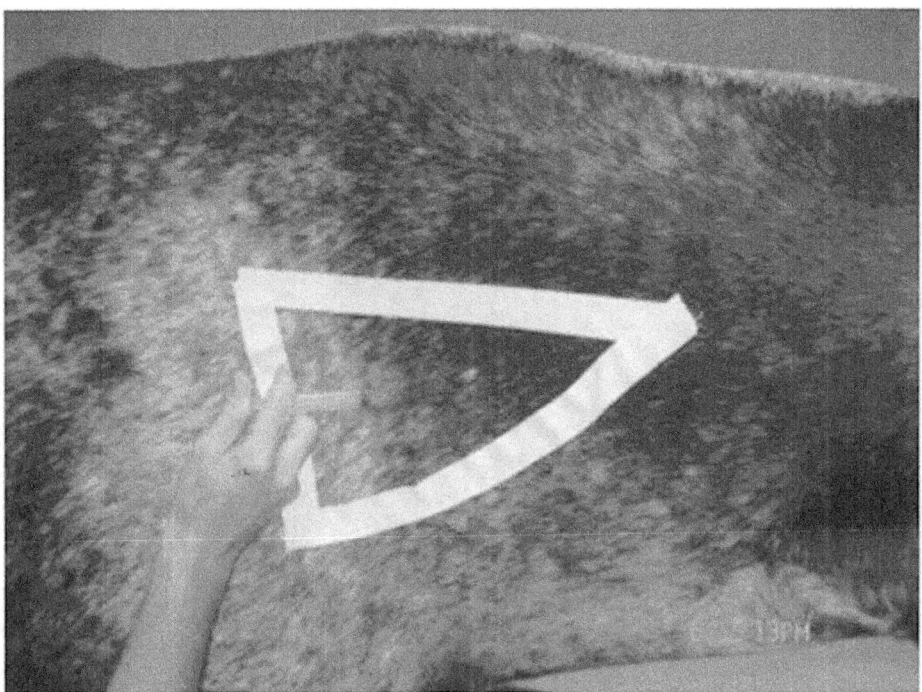

**Figure 3.1b:** *Proper Injection Technique*

## Buttocks (Gluteals) and Hind end (back of thigh)

Whenever repeated injections are needed, as in the case of antibiotic treatments, it is a good idea to alternate injections between all available sites. The rear end is a good area for injections, especially if a large volume injection (>10cc) is needed. Be sure to stand close to the horse's side and bump or tap the area with the ball of your hand to prepare the horse for receiving the needle. A major disadvantage to using the hind end is the risk of being kicked. Also if the site of injection were to have a reaction or develop an infection, the drainage on top of the buttocks is poor.

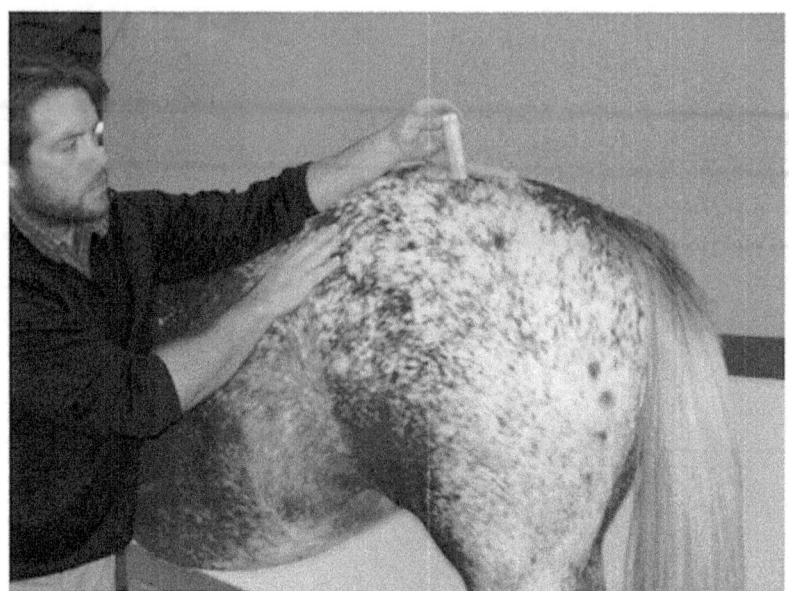

**Figure 3.2a:** *Intramuscular injection in the gluteals*

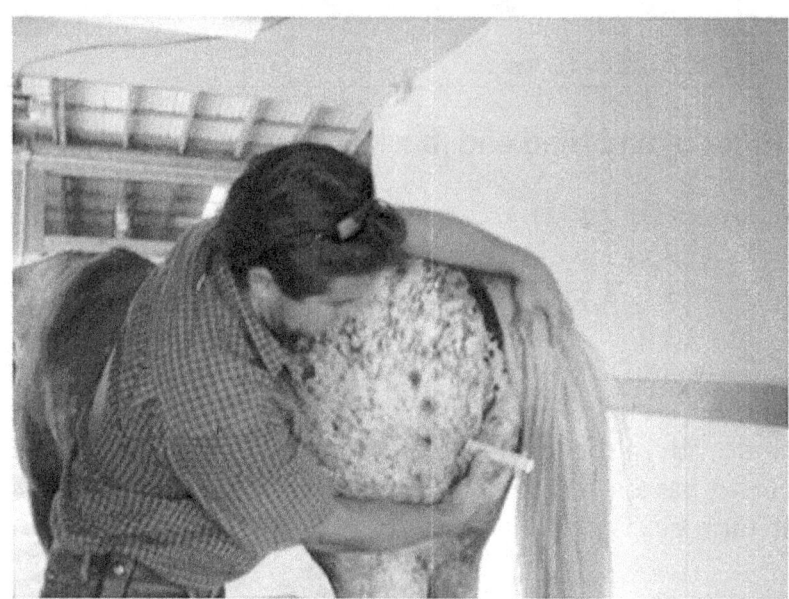

**Figure 3.2b:** *Intramuscular injection in the hind end*

## Chest

The chest is another area for the handler to give an IM injection. It is a bit more awkward than using the neck since the person giving the injection has to lean over and somewhat under the front of the horse. Be sure to stand to the side of the horse. I only use the chest if the other areas are too sore from repeated injections.

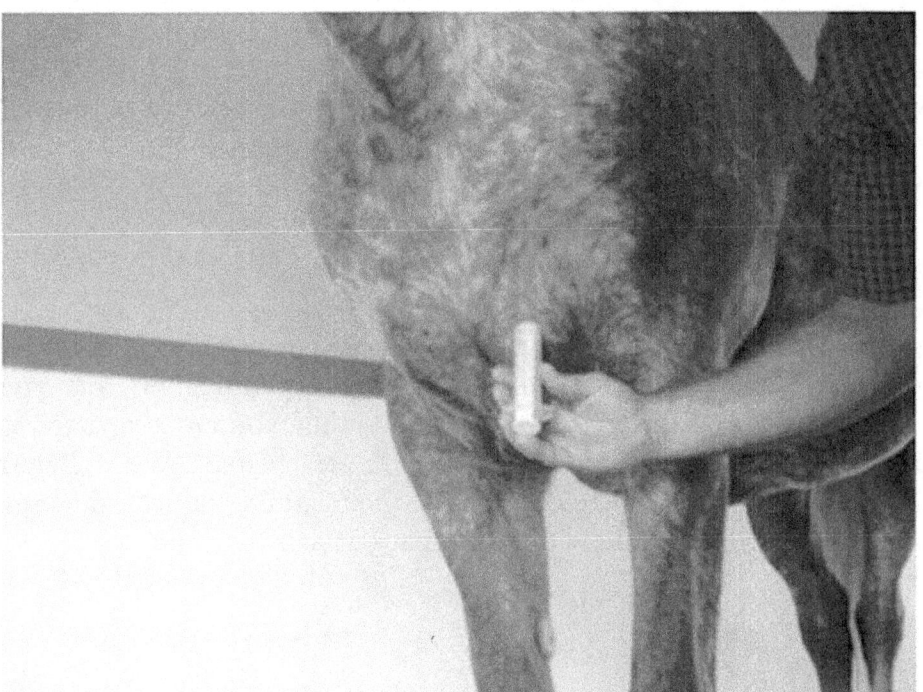

**Figure 3.3:** *IM injection in the chest*

As always, discuss all of the above vaccines with your veterinarian to decide which ones and at what intervals are appropriate for your horses. Vaccinating your horse on a regular basis not only keeps your horse healthier but it also allows you and your horse to develop a good working relationship with your veterinarian. If your veterinarian is checking your horse on a semi-annual basis, they can pick up on any subtle changes and perform regular dental exams while there.

On rare occasions anaphylactic vaccine reactions do occur and can be life threatening to your horse. Having a veterinarian there with the appropriate antidotes can mean the difference between life and death. Additionally, there are some vaccine manufacturers that provide a sort of insurance to horse owners that perform routine vaccination and de-worming for their horses. Basically, if all the guidelines are met, the company will provide financial assistance for the treatment of the horse if they were to contract one of the diseases they were vaccinated against. Consult with your veterinarian about these new programs.

Now that we have given you our guidelines on how to appropriately vaccinate your horse we can move on to de-worming principles for your animals.

## Deworming

In this section, we will summarize the most current concepts involving parasite control. Once again, it can vary depending on the type of situation your horse is in, the type of discipline you are associated with, and the area of the country in which you are located. We will start by covering each parasite individually, then anthelmintics, deworming schedules, and wrap it up with a summary of daily worming.

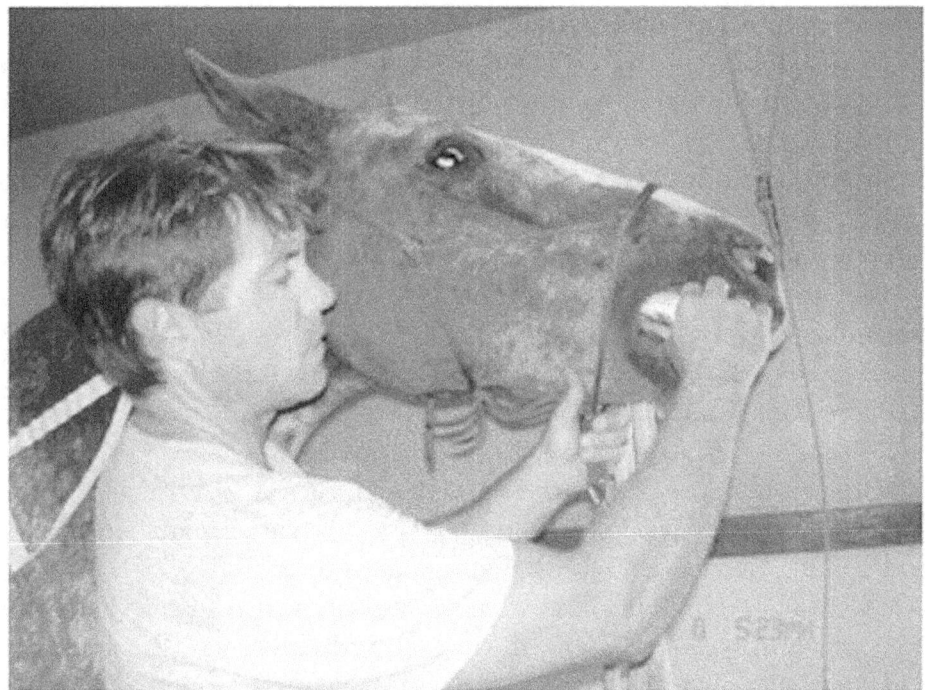

**Figure 3.4:** *Delivering Oral Medication*

## Defining a parasite

A parasite is an organism that lives within or on a host. It maintains its life and continues its life cycle with the help, or sometimes at the expense, of the host. This section on parasitology will be limited to worms, lice, ticks, flies, mites, and mosquitoes. There are plenty of other parasites out there, such as EPM and Potomac Horse Fever that horse owners should be aware of, but this section is limited to the discussion of those more common organisms recognized above.

Parasites differ from bacteria and viruses in a number of ways. Therefore, the prevention and control of parasites differs from that of bacteria and viruses. For example, many viral diseases can be vaccinated against and bacterial diseases are treated with the appropriate antibiotic. Unfortunately, animals do not build up immunity to parasites.

The majority of parasites are actually classified in the animal kingdom as animals. Therefore, in most cases they will have a lifecycle that requires them to leave their host to reproduce. Some of these lifecycles are quite complex and some have yet to be determined. The parasite's lifecycle is important to understand when it comes to controlling the parasite's replication and spread to your horse. For example, the elimination of standing or stagnant water can significantly reduce mosquito populations by ridding their breeding grounds. Composting of manure before spreading will raise the internal temperature thereby killing the eggs and parasites shed in the feces. The cleaner the environment, the less exposure your horse will have.

Many internal parasites today are resistant to de-wormers that were effective 15 years ago. Over time, parasites can mutate and become resistant to medical therapies that once were effective. Performing a fecal egg count can determine what type of burden your horse may have. Now we can focus our attention on each individual parasite and explore in greater detail how each one can affect your horse.

## Tapeworms (flatworm)

This is what I refer to as the new worm on the block! For years researchers felt that tapeworms were insignificant and caused little or no disease to the horse. However, research has developed in recent years concerning this parasite, leading to new de-wormers to treat tapeworm infestation. It is now believed that tapeworms occur much more frequently than first thought and that they can cause unique forms of colic. In the United States it is estimated that roughly 50-60% of horses are infected with some form of tapeworms. Like most parasites, in order to continue its lifecycle, it must return to the environment and be ingested by an oribatid mite, which are abundant in most horse pastures.

Based on the seasonal presence of the mite it is recommended that you de-worm for tapeworms on an early-Spring/late-Fall schedule. Another factor with tapeworms is the trouble in diagnostics for this worm. Often a regular fecal exam will not show tapeworms even though they are present in the digestive tract. A possible early sign associated with tapeworms may be diarrhea, especially in older horses. It is a good idea to incorporate a de-wormer effective against tapeworms in your de-worming program no matter what part of the country you.

## Ascarids (roundworms)

This is a group of worms that can infect a wide variety of mammalian species. Generally speaking they tend to be host-specific and will not transmit between species. That is, a roundworm specific for horses will not infect a dog or cat even if the animal is exposed. Ascarids tend to be unique in that they most often infect foals and yearlings and leave the adult animals alone even though they may be exposed.

The signs to look for in an infected animal are rough haircoat, pot-bellied appearance, lethargy, and possibly colic. Another sign that may be present during the migratory phase could be a mild cough.

The female ascarid worm is a prolific egg layer, and can produce literally millions of eggs in her lifetime. The egg is also resistant to environmental pressures, such as drying, cold and heat. Put all that together and you have a parasite that can be hard to control in a young growing animal's environment! When deworming for ascarids in a young animal that has a high burden, an impaction of dead worms can occur in the gut. Discuss with your veterinarian the use of a wormer that will not eradicate the worms all in one step. Using Panancur™ at half the recommended label dose for foals tends to remove roughly half of the worms, allowing one to repeat the process a week or two later at the full dosage. Controlling the amount of egg burden in the environment is an important part of the battle. If the contamination level in the environment is kept to a bare minimum then the animal is less likely to be infected.

## Strongyles

This is by far the most important and costly parasite you will deal with when treating your horse. Strongyles are divided into two different categories, large and small strongyles. Over the past several years, equine de-wormers have been successful and the strongyles have become rare in the environment. In some cases of well managed farms, large strongyles do not exist.

On the other hand, small strongyles are continuing to cause problems for horses and owners alike. This is primarily due to their ability to mutate and become ever resistant to modern de-wormers. Another characteristic that helps them survive even in the face of treatment is their ability to encyst in the intestinal lining to maintain viability in any situation and regardless of environmental pressures.

Though not too much trouble in young animals, this is by far the most debilitating and prolific parasite affecting adult horses. This is why most de-worming protocols discussed in this book will focus on controlling small strongyles.

## Bots (Gasterophilus sp.)

This is one of the few pests associated with horses that are transferred internally and can cause considerable GI damage to the host. The characteristic life cycle of the Bot fly includes a larval stage where the adult female fly deposits them on the skin of the horse to later be ingested when scratched off. These flies will be noticed in the late summer and early fall months. You may mistake them for a bee because the females make a buzzing sound as well as having a striped abdomen.

After depositing her eggs on the horse's hair (especially lower legs), the horse inadvertently ingests the newly hatched larvae. The larvae then migrate into the stomach region were they grow into adults, with each individual bot having a life span of up to a year. The extensive migration process and the lengthy life-span make it a potentially damaging parasite. It is also believed that these chronic lesions can create a life-time of GI problems for any animal if not addressed on a regular basis. Just like ascarids, environmental control is important to keep the worm burden low. By using a variety of external grooming tools, you can eliminate the parasite as its source. We use a pumice block that can be purchased from most feed or gardening stores. Keep in mind as well that modern dewormers geared toward bot protection are still quite effective.

## Other Parasites

This section will briefly cover a few minor parasites to keep in mind when developing your parasite control program. The first one is the threadworm, which is similar to ascarids in that it only affects young animals. The transmission from dam to foal via the milk is why the parasite is only seen in foals aged 1-5 months. Another aspect that makes this parasite unique is that most animals have developed immunity to this parasite by 6 months of age.

The next parasite is pinworms. This worm has a distinctive life-cycle in that the adult does not discharge her eggs in the manure, but migrates to the rectal area and sticks her eggs to the perineal area. This is the parasite most responsible for tail rubbing. Modern de-wormers can effectively control pinworms when used properly.

There a few other groups of parasites to mention and they include stomach worms, lung worms, and skin worms. If using appropriate modern de-wormers, you can control all of these parasites.

Now that we know what parasites we are fighting, the next section will cover which de-wormers are right for each individual type of parasite.

# Anthelmintics

Anthelmintics is a fancy word for de-wormer. A de-wormer is a medical preparation used to treat and kill parasites in animals. Over the years, several de-wormers have been used effectively, and for the vast majority of them with little side effects. The biggest challenge with de-wormers today is parasite resistance. This is why new de-wormers are constantly being improved and new de-worming protocols are being identified.

The next sections breakdown each individual de-wormer and explore its effectiveness and possible side effects.

## Pyrantal pamoate/tartrate (Strongid™)

This class of de-wormers is effective safe to the environment. It is used most often in juvenile animals to help primarily in the treatment of ascarids. Although not effective against the larvacidal stage, it is effective against the adult stage of the ascarid.

Another important use for Strongid™ is the treatment of tapeworms. If dosed three times the normal dose, Strongid™ is effective against tapeworms. This is generally done via tubing the animal and using a dose syringe to administer.

Strongid™ is also the ingredient found in the daily wormer. The daily wormer is a pelleted product intended to be fed to your horse on a daily basis. The jury is still out as to the benefits of this product. In our experience it seems to keep the animal looking and feeling healthier. However there has been some evidence to suggest an increased amount of parasite resistance to Strongid™, when used on a regular basis.

## Fenbendazole (Panacur™ or Safegard™)

This class of de-wormer, although effective, seems to have the most trouble with parasite resistance. That is why the company that produces this product has marketed it as an extended product. It seems that if used at a higher dose for three consecutive days or at the regular dose for five consecutive days, the effectiveness increases. Although this sounds expensive, when compared to some of the other de-wormers, it is by far one of the safest ones on the market for any age animal. It can also be dosed in a paste or liquid preparation. This is important for large operations that prefer to use a dose gun when worming large numbers of animals at a time.

### Ivermectin (Eqvalan™, Zimecterin™, etc.)

This is the most well known and currently one of the most effective de-wormers on the market today. Aside from being so effective, it is also broad spectrum. From ascarids to strongyles and all the parasites in between, it kills them with the same effectiveness. The only parasite that seems to be immune is the tapeworm. This de-wormer, like fenbendazole, is also available in a liquid preparation to be used in a gun de-wormer.

### Moxidectin (Quest™)

Quest™ is in the same category as Ivermectin, in that it is an effective de-wormer against a wide variety of parasites. The only difference is that Quest™ seems to have a narrow dosing margin and it can cause a wide variety of side effects. Make sure that you are accurate when estimating your horse's weight and dose accordingly. You will want to use caution when using in young animals or miniature horses. However, if dosed accurately, this can be one of the more effective de-wormers used in equine medicine today.

### Praziquantel

This is a newer de-worming preparation on the block. The actual drug has been used for years in dogs and cats. It is used in the treatment of tapeworms. Praziquantel can be found formulated with either Ivermectin or Moxidectin. Overall this is an effective and safe product.

## To Rotate or Not?

Now that we have covered the most prevalent parasites and the modern day de-wormers that can be used, it is time to formulate a parasite program. Currently the idea is to rotate de-wormers on an every other month basis, and to de-worm every animal with the same intensity. However, due to new research, it may not be advisable to continue de-worming in this fashion. The current thought is that de-worming every animal on a regular basis may cause an increase in parasite resistance. It is now recommended that a fecal egg count be performed on every animal, and then the ones with high egg counts be de-wormed accordingly.

Check with your veterinarian to see if they have the facilities to perform the egg count or can send the sample off to a local lab. The money spent on doing a thorough diagnostic work-up can save you money in unnecessary de-wormers for horses who do not need to be treated. Keep in mind that, at this time, there are no new de-wormers under development. There could be trouble ahead if the parasites continue to become resistant to the current de-wormers.

## The Preventicare Program

This is a program developed by a manufacturing company called Pfizer™. The idea is that if you maintain your horse's vaccination, de-worming, and dental program on a regular basis, your horse will be healthier and at less risk of colic. With the help of your veterinarian, you must first fill out an application for each of your horses and then start them on daily Strongid™ therapy. If your horses qualify and continue with the program's requirements, you will be reimbursed $5,000 towards the expense of colic surgery at an approved facility. Investigate this program with your vet and see if it would work for your animals.

The importance of having a Coggins Test done on a regular basis will wrap up the topics for this chapter.

# The Coggin's Test

The Coggin's test was developed about forty years ago by a veterinarian named Dr. Bob Coggins. It is used to test for an incurable disease called Equine Infectious Anemia (EIA). This disease is spread via biting flies such as horse flies and deer flies.

Once a horse contracts the disease, their immune system becomes impaired and over a period of time is destroyed to the point that the animal dies. The worst part of equine infectious anemia is that there is no treatment or prevention for the disease at this time. Because of the destructive nature of this disease, the test was developed to check horses on a yearly basis and make sure they are negative. This is essential when animals congregate at a show or trail ride so that the disease will not be spread. If an animal is infected, the course of action is lifetime quarantine or euthanasia. All things considered, that is why it is so vital to have your horse tested on an annual basis. In North Carolina there is legislation that will impose stiff fines for offenders.

## Quarantine

From vaccination to de-worming, you can now understand how important it can be to quarantine all new animals coming on to your property. This can help keep the incidence of disease low at your facilities. It can also give you time to check the animal's preventative care program to date and modify it if needed. One item to make sure of is that the horse has a negative Coggin's test.

## Conclusion

From vaccination to de-worming, the proper preventative program for your horse is the core of equine health. By incorporating these important aspects of equine life into your horse program, your horses will maintain an overall healthier life. As always discuss any of these ideas and suggestions with your veterinarian so you can establish the right program for all your horses.

We have stressed above how important it is to look at each individual animal because the recommendations will most likely be different for each one. It is our hope that by following these simple ideals, the incidence of emergencies you encounter will remain low due to your dedication to prevention. Not all accidents can be prevented, so read on to gain more important knowledge in the event your horse does require emergency care.

# Reproductive Emergencies – The Pregnant Mare

CHAPTER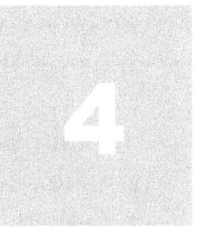

Now that we have a better understanding of what an emergency truly is and all the intricate parts associated with one, it is time to break them down on an individual basis and learn more about them. What better category to start with than reproductive emergencies. Just like in human medicine, this area can be one of the most frustrating aspects of veterinary medicine to manage. Once you think you are an expert at dealing with pregnant mares, one will come along and fool you. This section will encompass reproductive emergencies only, and then we will break the neonatal emergencies down in the next chapter. This chapter begins with an explanation of what is normal followed by some emergency situations you may encounter.

## Normal Gestation

The normal gestation period for a mare is between 320 and 365 days. On average this is 338 days. This varies with the breed of horse as well. A foal born before 320 days is considered premature, which can be cause of great concern to the health of the foal. However, foaling late does not seem to be as wrought with complications. We have even seen mares carry their foal for a whole year. Once again, it is essential to keep accurate records on your mare so that you can be aware of any abnormalities. You can then compare them from previous pregnancies to check for any trends in your mare's gestation history. This can help if your mare tends to have premature foals, then you can be prepared if needed.

It is very important to have your mare checked in foal at about 14-16 days to deal with the possibility of the occurrence of a twinning. If your mare has produced twins, this is the critical time in which that problem can be resolved. This is accomplished by manually collapsing one of the embryos, thus terminating one pregnancy to save the other.

Maintain an adequate level of nutrition for the expectant mother and normalcy in her every day routine. Remember to take your mare off endophyte fescue hay and pasture three months before parturition. This will eliminate her or the foal from suffering the deleterious side effects of the endophyte in some fescue hays and pastures. Have the proper facilities available for your mare to give birth. This will help keep the new foal warm and dry, no matter when it is born.

You will need to vaccinate your mare against Equine Herpes Virus - Type 1 (EHV-1) with a product such as Pneumobort-K at the fifth, seventh, and ninth month. In some endemic areas you may need to start at 3 months. This will help prevent the chance of your mare aborting her foal if she contracts this particular rhinovirus during gestation. It is highly recommended that you vaccinate your mare for Eastern Equine Encephalitis (EEE), Western Equine Encephalitis (WEE), Flu, Rhino, Tetanus, Rabies and West Nile in the last 4-6 weeks of parturition to help boost the antibodies in the colostrum. Then when the foal nurses the antibody rich colostrum, his immune system should develop effectively.

## Education

In many areas, your county extension service or universities may offer short 1-2 day classes that can give you a wealth of information. This will improve your confidence while caring for your pregnant mare. Your veterinarian can also give you information that together with this handbook will enable you to solve many minor problems that may arise. To cover this topic we will use a chronological approach form the moment your mare conceives until she foals.

# Breeding Emergencies

To preface this following section, we are not attempting to describe all the steps involved with breeding management. That is another topic entirely. We will address only aspects surrounding breeding that are or could lead to an emergency. Today, most people hand breed or artificially inseminate their mares in order to decrease the chance of accidents occurring and for convenience. The old saying, an ounce of prevention is worth a pound of cure, applies here so save some grief by being careful. When hand-breeding, caution is needed to protect the mare and the stallion, and more importantly the people. Stallions can suffer severe injury when mounting a mare that kicks. Hobbles and/or a twitch for the mare may be necessary. In rare cases, the mare may need some mild sedation if she is nervous or aggressive. First, we will address a couple of stallion emergencies.

## Stallions

### Paraphimosis

This is the fancy term for the inability of your stallion or gelding to retract his penis into his sheath. The primary cause is usually trauma to the penis with resultant swelling and sometimes nerve damage. It can result when a mare kicks the stallion's penis. Other causes may include spinal injuries, inflammation secondary to sedation, or viral infection and edema of the prepuce secondary to castration, just to name a few. It is very important to have this evaluated by your veterinarian immediately.

### Treatment

**Reduce Swelling**- In the early stages, use cool water therapy. This can be accomplished using water or ice. Most horses tend to tolerate cold-hosing pretty well. After the acute phase, alternate with cold and warm therapy.

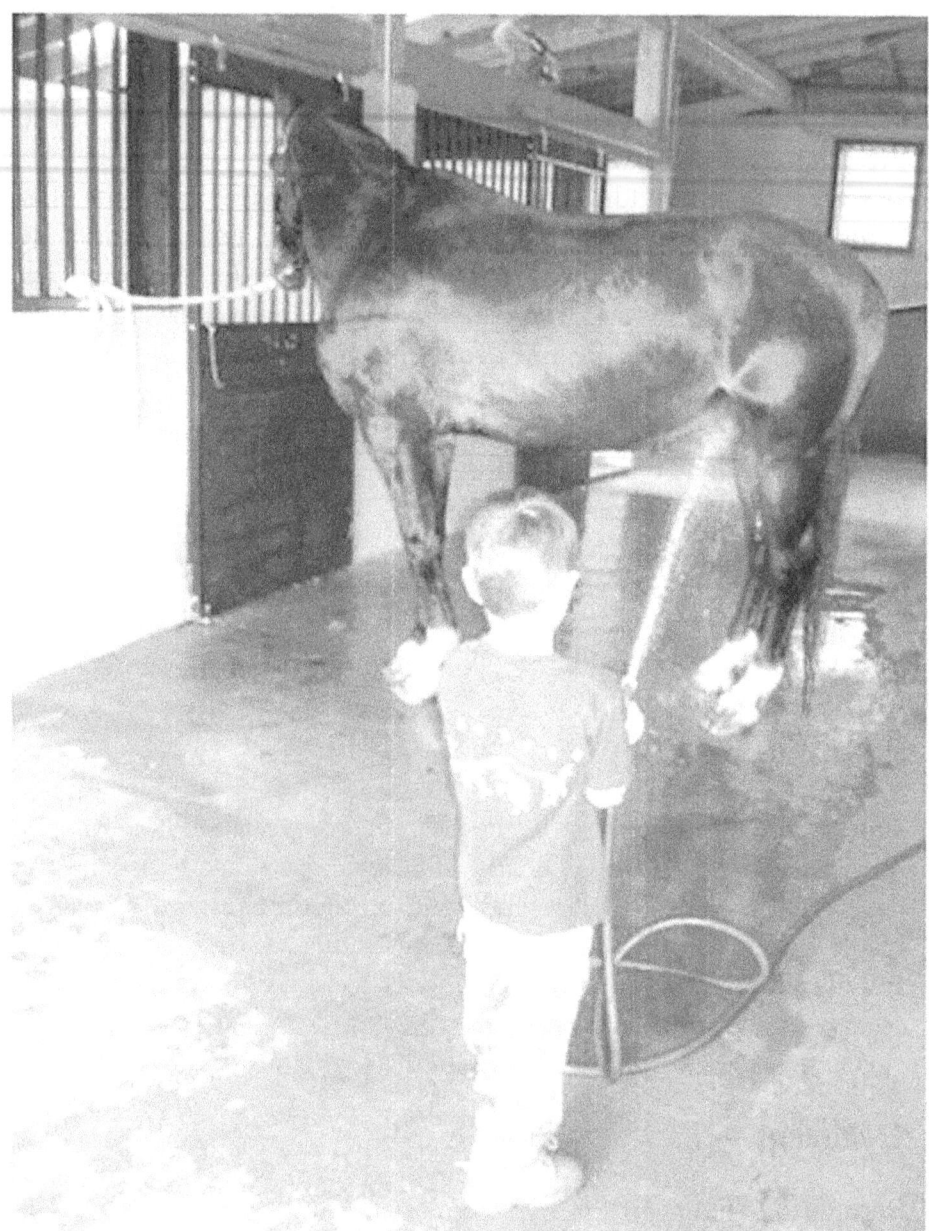

Figure 4.1: *Cold-hosing Sheath*

**Support**- Prevent the penis from being further damaged by providing some support or a sling. We have used old bed sheets to keep the penis close to the belly wall. Remember that gravity is working against you in a vicious cycle.

**Cleanse**- Keep the penis clean using a mild cleanser such as Ivory soap™. Make sure to rinse the penis completely.

**Antibiotics or lubricants**- You may also have to apply some topical antibiotic therapy or lubricants such as Vaseline™ and hand creams to dry and cracked areas. Wait to do this until your veterinarian examines it first.

Your veterinarian may tell you to give a dose of flunixin or bute to get a head start with the swelling before they arrive.

## Penile Hematoma

This occurs when a stallion gets kicked directly on his erect penis when breeding a mare or some other unwilling horse. The trauma then causes an enormous blood clot to occur in the penile area. The treatment for this emergency is very similar to the one above. It is important to keep the swelling to a minimum from the start. Start by cold hosing the area with water, and consult your veterinarian to see if they want you to initiate anti-inflammatory therapy prior to their arrival.

## Scrotal hernia

A scrotal hernia happens when internal abdominal structures pass through the inguinal rings into the scrotal sac. I have seen this occur in one stallion post-breeding; however, it can occur at times unrelated to breeding. Fortunately, this condition is uncommon. You will see swelling in the scrotum, often only on one side. In short, this is an emergency surgery situation. The tissues entrapped in the scrotum may contain bowel (intestines) which can be strangled from their blood supply in a short period of time. Your vet will most likely refer you to a surgical facility for immediate care. A dose of anti-inflammatory medication may be necessary during transit as this condition can be quite painful.

# Mares

## Vaginal Bleeding

If you see blood coming from the vagina after breeding, try to assess how much bleeding is actually occurring. In some maiden mares you will see a small amount of bleeding from rupturing the hymen, which is the thin membrane inside vagina, during the first breeding. This is normal and will pass without incident. If this is not a maiden mare and/or the bleeding is severe or continues for more than 5-10 minutes, consult with your veterinarian. They may want to do a digital exam to determine the source of the bleeding and what extent of damage has occurred. In the meantime, cease all breeding activity and try to keep the mare calm and quiet in a stall with hay. Monitor the mucous membranes and capillary refill time. Refer to Chapter 1 for information on this topic.

## Rectal Bleeding

This is a life threatening problem. It can occur when the stallion enters rectally instead of vaginally. Rectal tears are graded from 1-4 depending upon the depth of the tear in the rectal wall tissue. Many horses die from rectal tears secondary to septic shock if the bowel contents start spilling into the sterile abdominal cavity. Once the mare is examined your vet can make determinations as to the severity of the tear and whether the horse should be referred to a surgical facility. There are specialized breeding rolls that can be affixed under the mare's tail to help prevent this accident. The rolls may also be used when the stallions have excessively long penises and penetrate too deep. You should keep the mare quiet as with a vaginal tear until help arrives.

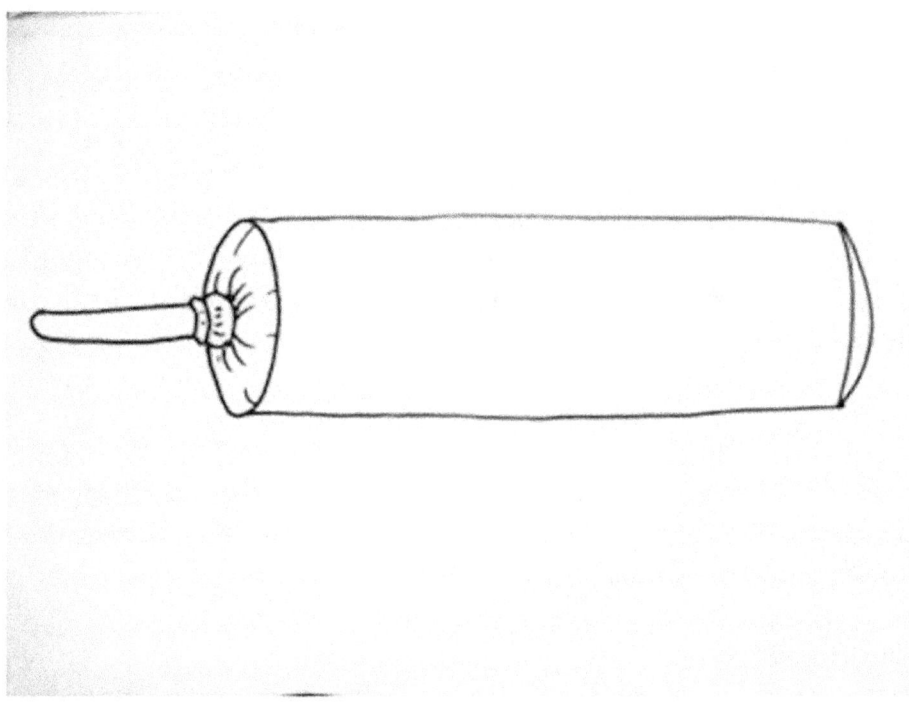

**Figure 4.2:** *Breeding roll*

## Abortion

Abortion is defined as the premature expulsion of a fetus during pregnancy. Abortion may be early, mid or late term. Oftentimes, early abortions may go unnoticed, and actually be completely resorbed inside the mare's uterus. In these cases no outward signs may be seen. However, mid to late term abortions can sometimes be preceded by signs of fever, discomfort, inappetance, vaginal discharge, and occasionally early lactation (milk production).

Abortions may be caused by placental infection (fungal/viral/bacterial), placental insufficiencies, twins, umbilical cord torsions, colic, toxins/poisons, or other systemic disease. I have actually been called to examine aborting mares that were forcibly hand bred to the stallion while they were pregnant! All cases resulted in abortion. You can alert your vet to the aforementioned signs to see if an exam is warranted to ensure fetal viability.

In some cases, antibiotics, hormones and other therapies can be administered in high-risk patients. If you happen to find your mare aborted without any warning signs, it is advised to collect the fetus and afterbirth, if it is not decomposed, place it in a trash bag, place the bag on ice, and submit to a veterinary diagnostic lab for testing. Blood samples may be collected from the mare to run tests for diseases related to abortion. Also have the mare cultured before breeding again to treat any possible uterine infection(s). If you have other mares in the same vicinity, remove them until contagions can be ruled out. As a reminder, vaccinate your mare against Equine Rhinopneumonitis, which is a disease caused by equine herpes virus Type 1 (EHV-1), during the 3rd, 5th, 7th, and 9th months of gestation.

## Placentitis

The placenta is an organ that serves as a lifeline between the mare and foal during pregnancy. Normal function is essential for a successful pregnancy. Early detachment or inflammation in the placenta could lead to abortion or premature birth. One sign to look for would be early udder development 1-2 months prior to foaling, along with lactation (milk leaking). Treatment with antibiotics and hormones is usually indicated once the diagnosis is made.

## Dystocia

Dystocia is difficulty that occurs when the mare is in labor. You (and your mare) have waited all year for the fateful day and tragedy strikes! On a more serious note, this problem can lead to the loss of mare and foal if not corrected immediately. If you have attended a foaling class or have experience with foaling before, you know that once mares are in active labor, it goes quickly, and the foal is often born in 30 minutes or less.

Powerful contractions from the mare exert tremendous pressure on the foal and birth canal. If the mare is in the final stages of labor and is straining without result for more than 10 minutes, chances are that something is wrong! If the foal is oversized or not positioned correctly, a normal birth will not occur. Even if you call your vet out and they arrive within the hour, sometimes it is too late to save the foal and attention is then diverted to saving the mare.

The placenta begins to detach at the onset of labor, thereby depriving the foal of oxygen if not delivered in sufficient time. Since you are in a situation where you need to act quickly, you may need to assist the mare by redirecting the foal into proper position for delivery before help can arrive. You stand to lose a lot more by doing nothing than by doing something.

There is serious risk of injury to human handlers while assisting a mare in dystocia. The mares are in extreme pain and can act without warning by kicking, turning, dropping to the ground, or rising suddenly. Do not put yourself in harm's way! I have coached many people over the phone while racing down the road in the middle of the night, but I always stress that their own physical safety is more important to me than the mare's safety. Above all remain calm and collected, since stress will only cloud your judgment!

Your foaling kit should have sterile lubricants (KY jelly™) in the event that you need to intervene in this manner. Sometimes all that is necessary is to extend one or both of the front legs into a diving position (hooves in front of the nose) to allow passage.

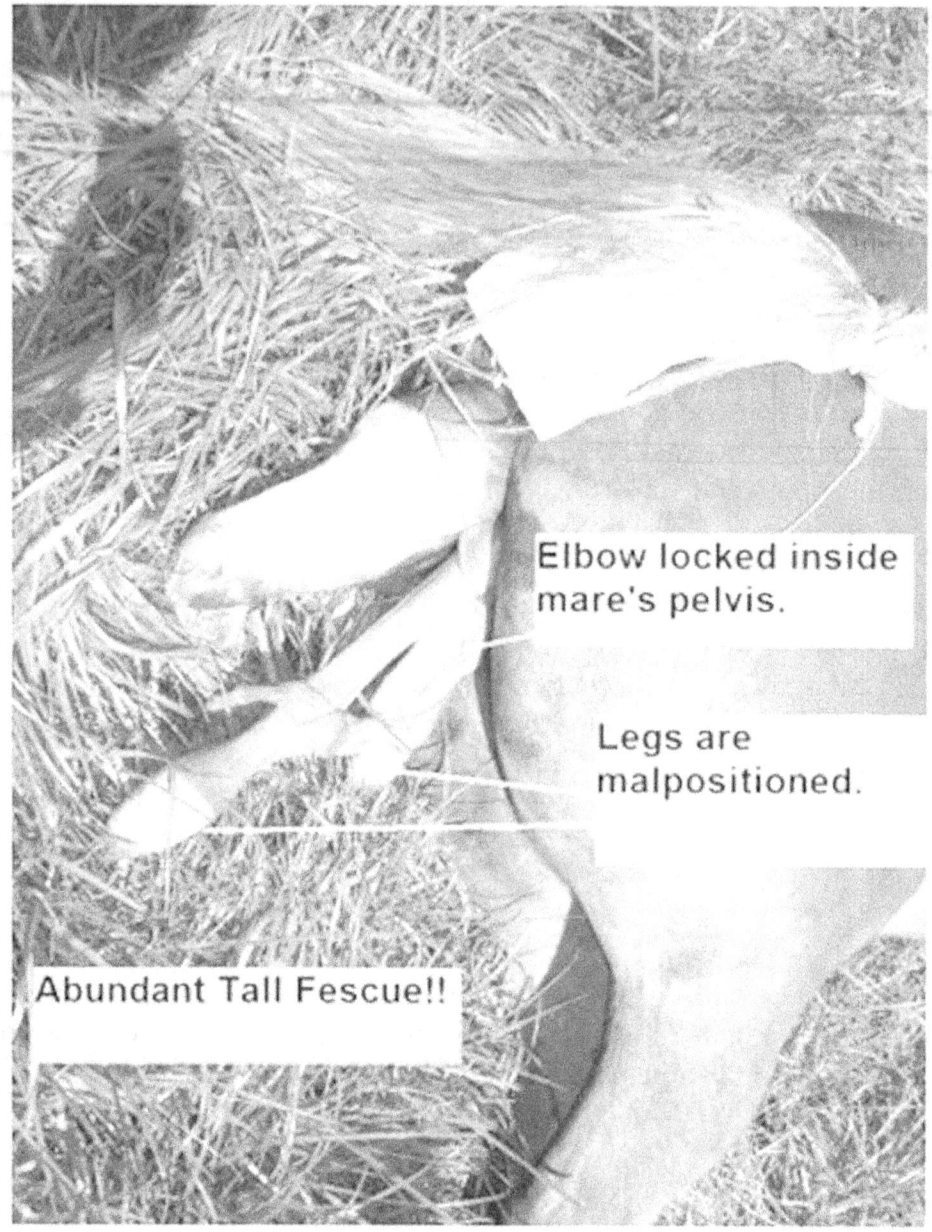

**Figure 4.3a:** *Dystocia--Elbow locked*

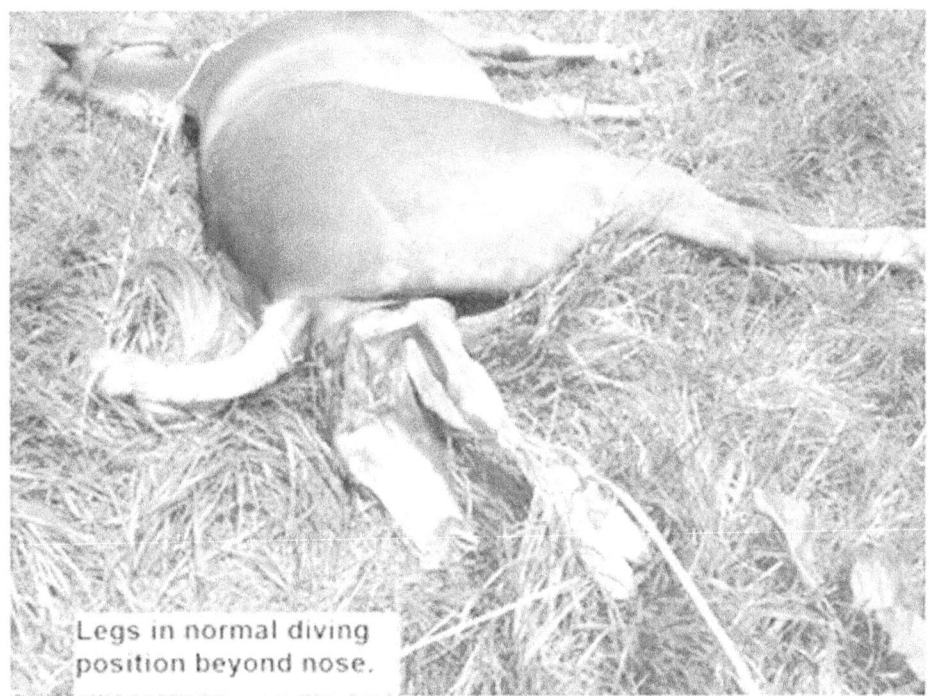

**Figure 4.3b**: *Dystocia corrected*

Unless you have previous experience, do not extend your hand into the mare's vagina more than a few inches. You could cause damage to the sensitive vaginal tissue. Clip fingernails if necessary! Also, the mare may be unpredictable since she may be in pain and harm you in the process. The powerful contractions can actually break bones (yours) if your arm is between the foal and mare's pelvis. Be careful! Sedation and an epidural (anesthetic nerve block to lower spine) performed by your vet is needed in most cases to ease the contractions and pain while adjustments and manipulations are made.

Open the whitish sac (amnion) that surrounds the foal before making manipulations. Also remove this sac from the foal's head as soon as the head and nostrils are presented. If you notice a prominent bulging at the mare's upper vagina or rectal area, immediately reach in and direct the foal's legs out to avoid tearing the mare's rectal-vaginal tissue.

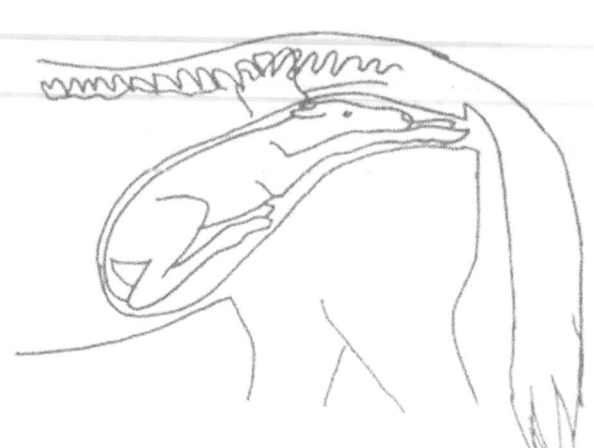

**Figure 4.4:** *Normal foaling position*

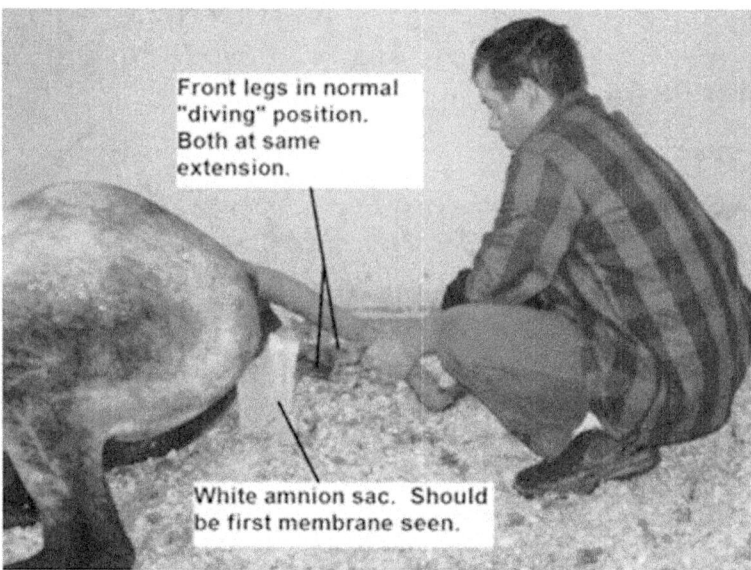

**Figure 4.5:** *Amnion and front legs normal*

When a foal is in the normal position, the front feet come first with the soles facing downward. If the foal is backward (hindlegs first) the soles will be facing up. In the backward position, there is added risk of early umbilical severance, thus depriving the foal of oxygen before the birth is complete. If you are in this situation, help the mare by pulling during the contractions. Be sure to pull in a downward direction (see illustration). Pulling straight out may cause the foal's hips to lock inside the mares pelvis. Remember to use plenty of lubrication to reduce any friction.

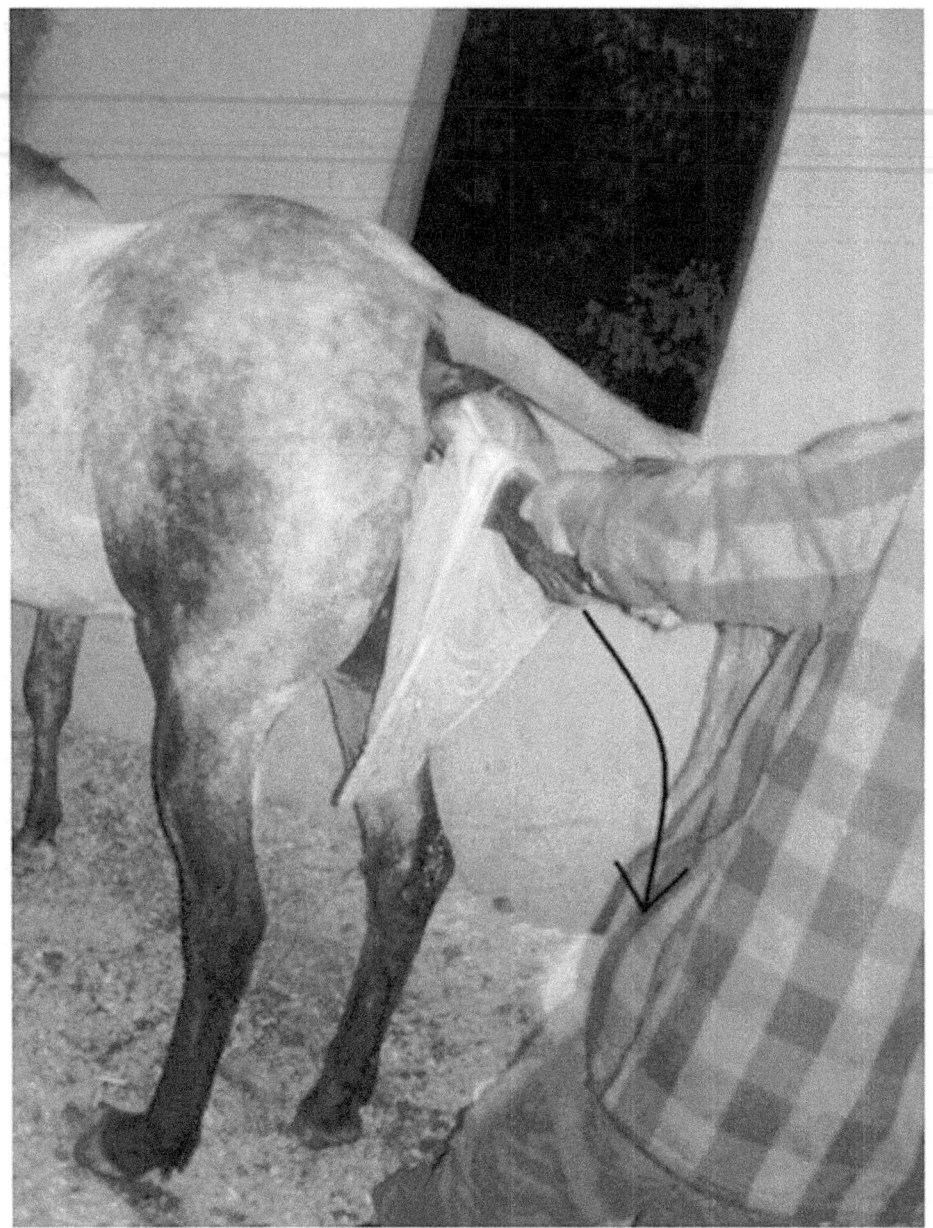

**Figure 4.6:** *Pull downward during contractions*

The following images depict other abnormal presentations.

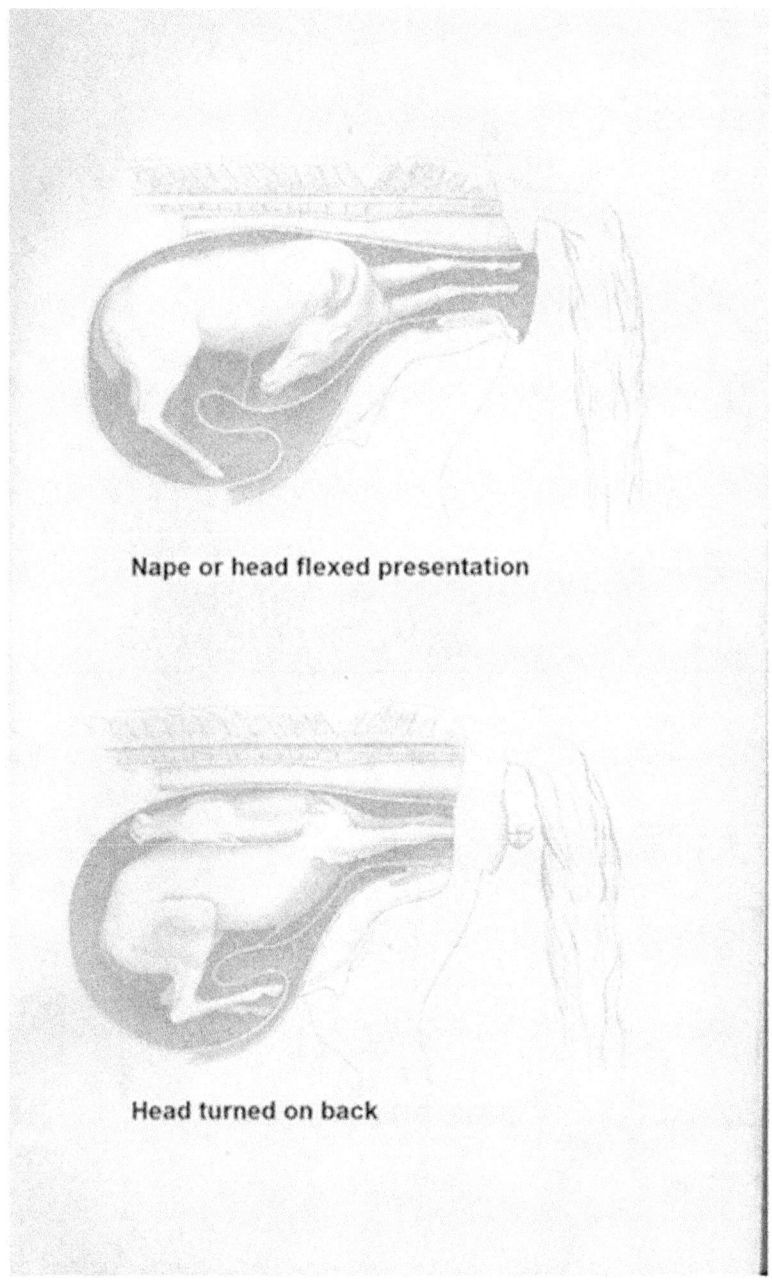

**Figure 4.7a:** *Abnormal presentations- Head flexed or turned*

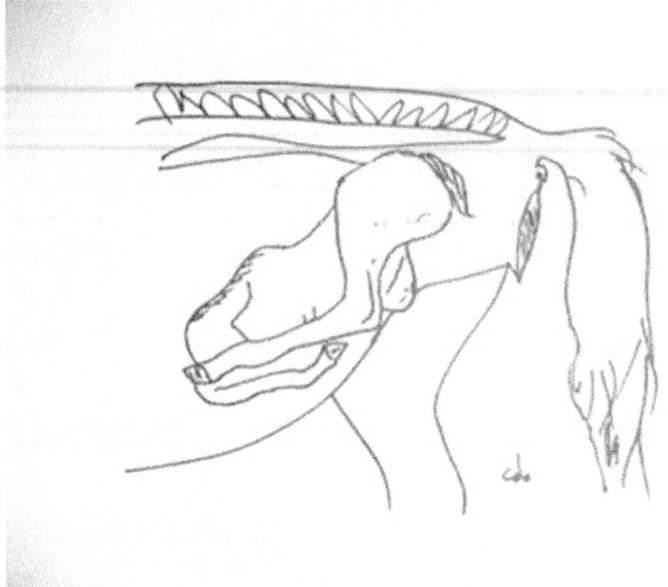

**Figure 4.7b:** *Abnormal presentation - Breech*

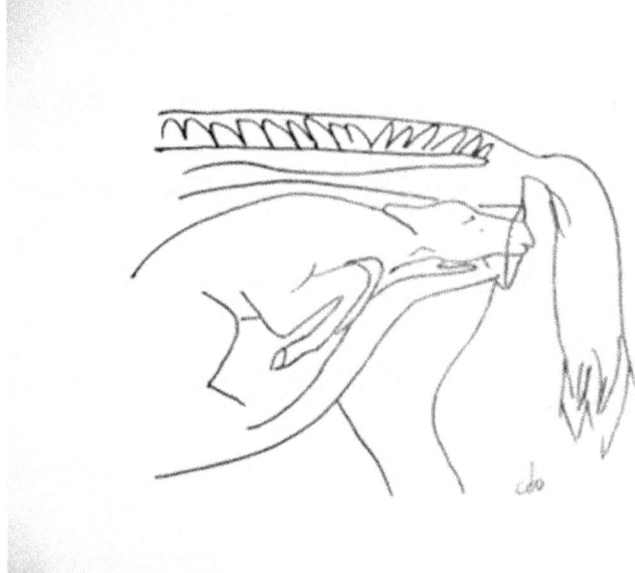

**Figure: 4.7c:** *Abnormal presentation - Carpal Flexion*

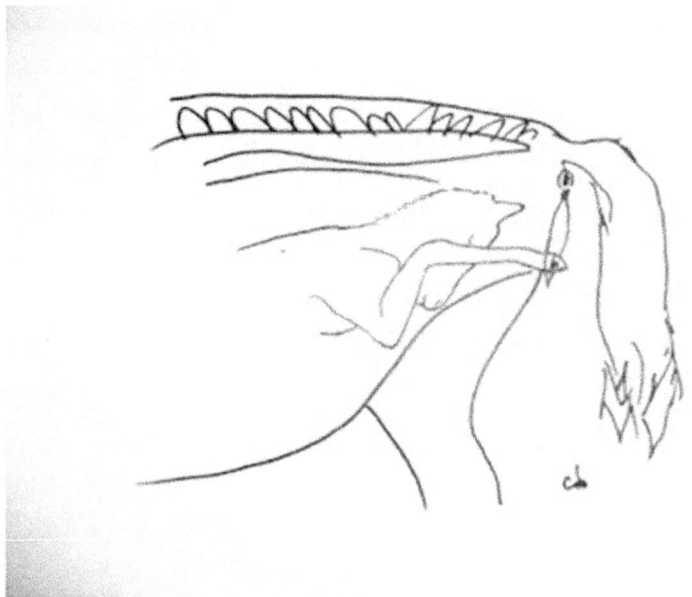

**Figure 4.7d:** *Abnormal presentation – Nape (poll first)*

Once the foal is successfully delivered, it should begin breathing and moving around. The umbilicus may still be attached. Do not disturb this connection. The umbilicus will naturally break when the mare or foal stands. If there is too much commotion or interference, the mare may get up too quickly and cause the cord to break prematurely. If there is apparent blood leaking from the navel, tie it off quickly and disinfect with 1 part chlorhexadine to 10 parts water as described in Chapter 2. The next chapter will get into more detail about the foal.

## Redbag (Placenta Previa)

This condition occurs when the placental sac fails to rupture. If you see a red sac protruding from the vagina instead of the normal glistening white sac of the amnion, immediately intervene. In other words, the "breaking of water" fails to occur while the placenta is detaching from the mare's uterus. This will present many problems. The foal's oxygen supply will be compromised because the connection of the uterus and the placenta is being lost while normal delivery is not occurring. The foal will not deliver out of the vaginal opening until the placenta ruptures, thus causing dystocia. You will need to manually rupture this sac if it appears from the vagina. Use your fingers to tear the sac open as soon as you notice it. A large amount of fluid should rush out. Normal delivery should commence immediately. If there is a question as to how long the mare has been in this condition, there may be a high risk for foal complications.

Normally these membranes will be expelled from the mare in the first hour after delivery. Gravity is usually all that is needed to help them pass. If a large portion of the membranes is hanging and touching the ground, take some twine and tie them up to around hock level.

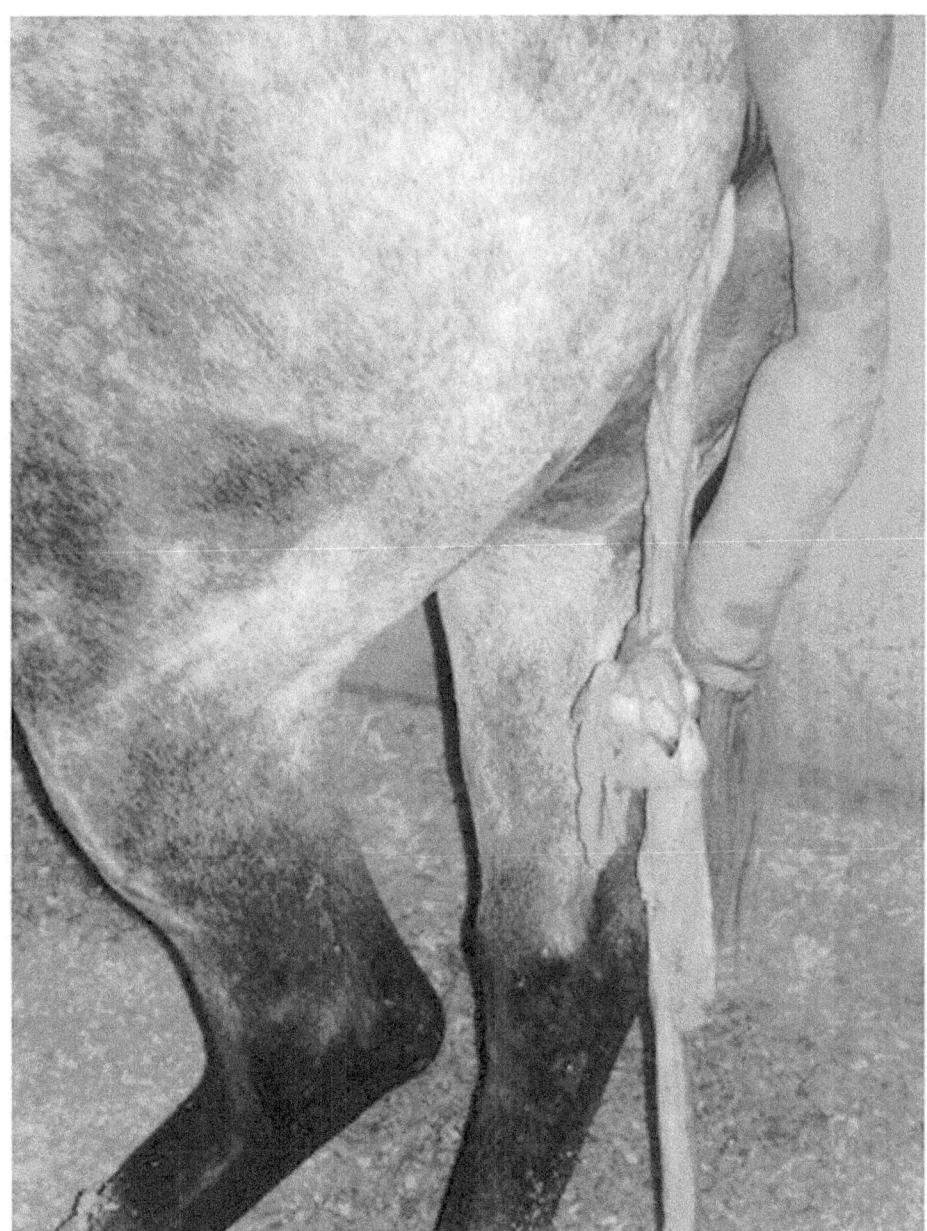

**Figure 4.8:** *Placenta tied in a knot*

Never try to pull the membranes out. If they are retained longer than 3 hours, assistance may be needed to remove them. The retained placenta can lead to systemic sickness if all or a portion is left inside the mare. The mare with a retained placenta is an emergency that should be corrected in the first 6-8 hours if possible.

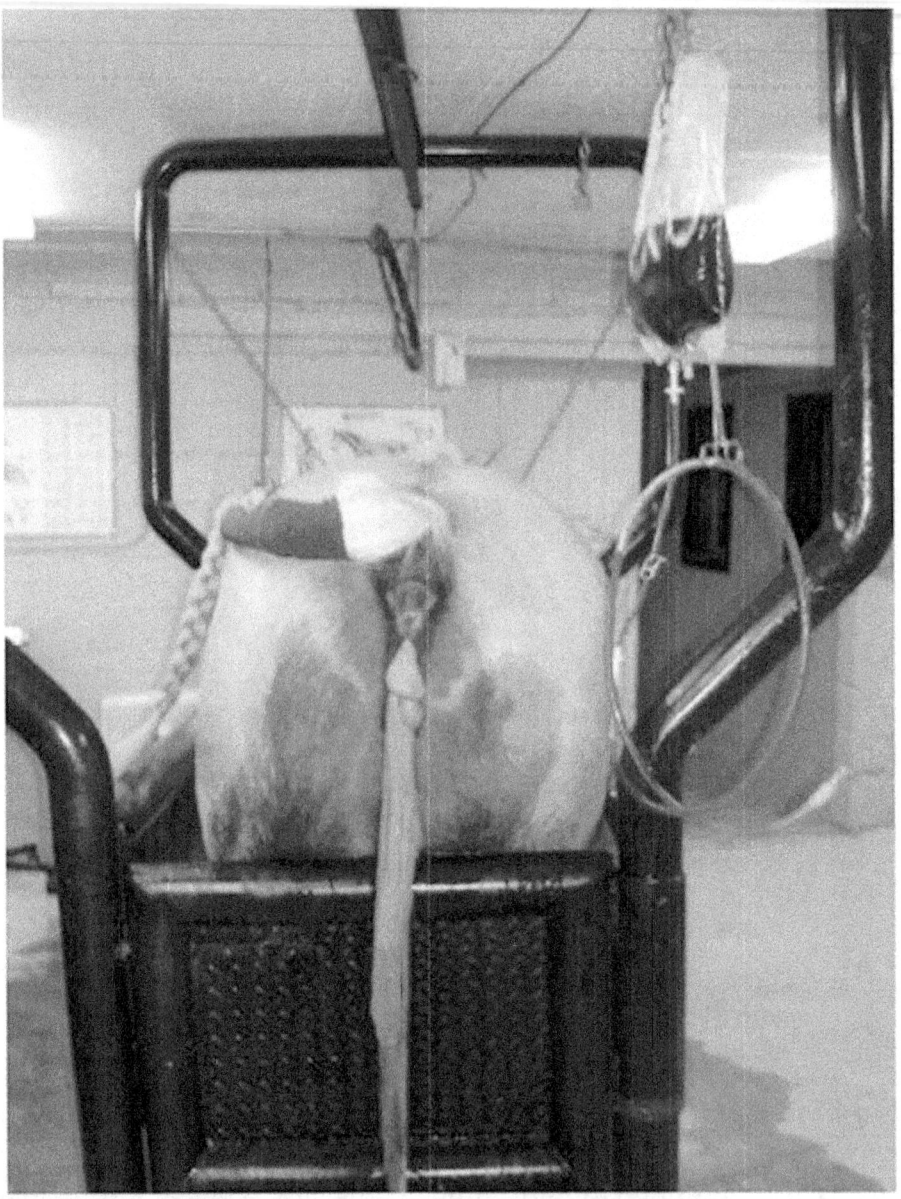

**Figure 4.7:** *Retained Placenta (afterbirth) prior to treatment*

Antibiotics and anti-inflammatory medication are necessary to counter the side effects of the dead membrane. Your veterinarian may carefully remove the placenta manually, or treat the mare with infusions/lavages to help the detachment. In all cases, you should have the after birth examined for completeness once it is expelled. Even if you don't see anything hanging from the mare's vulva, there could be a small remnant inside. If left untreated, some mares can founder, contract tetanus, or be left with damaged uterine lining thereby compromising future breeding.

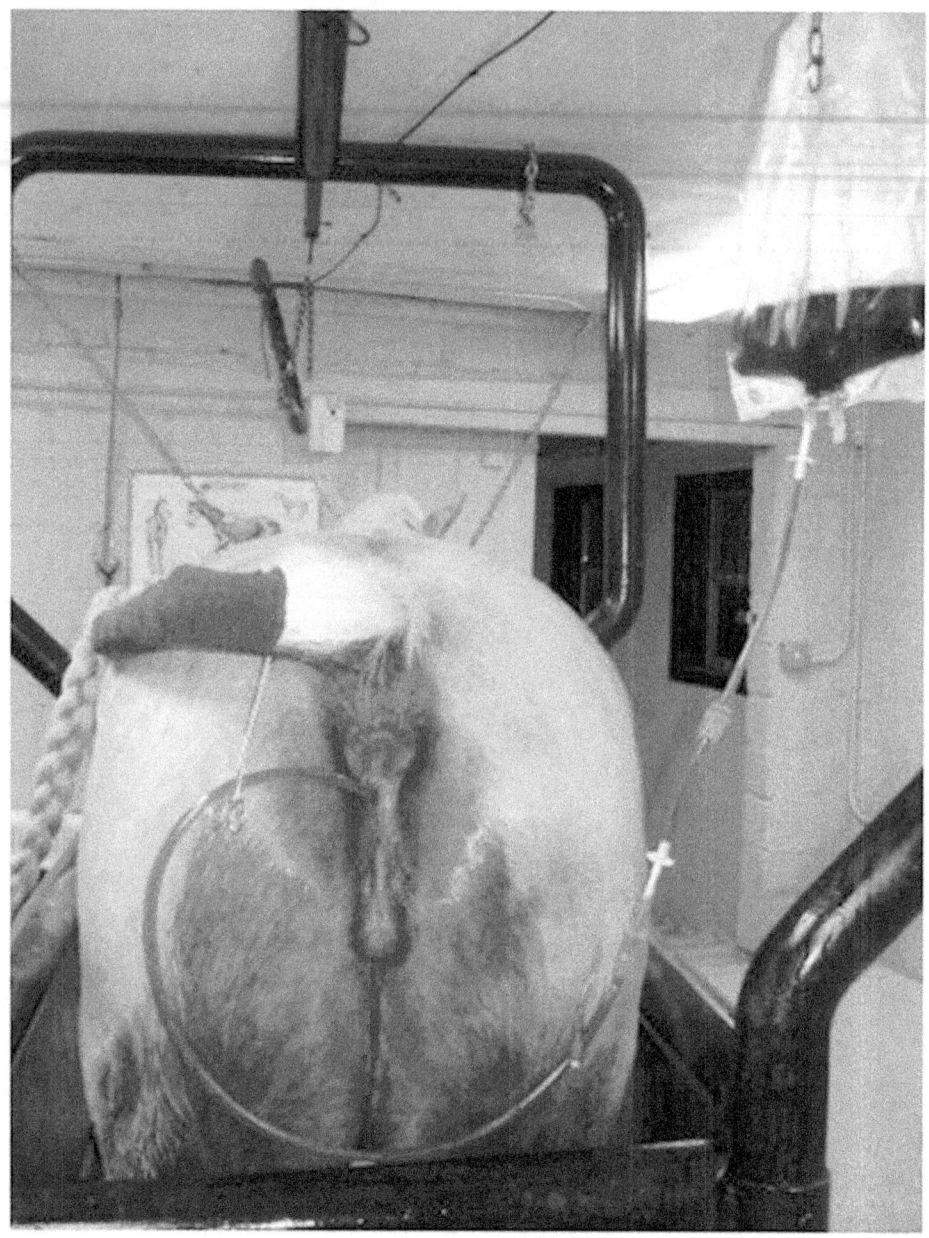

**Figure 4.8:** *Placenta passed after infusion and oxytocin therapy*

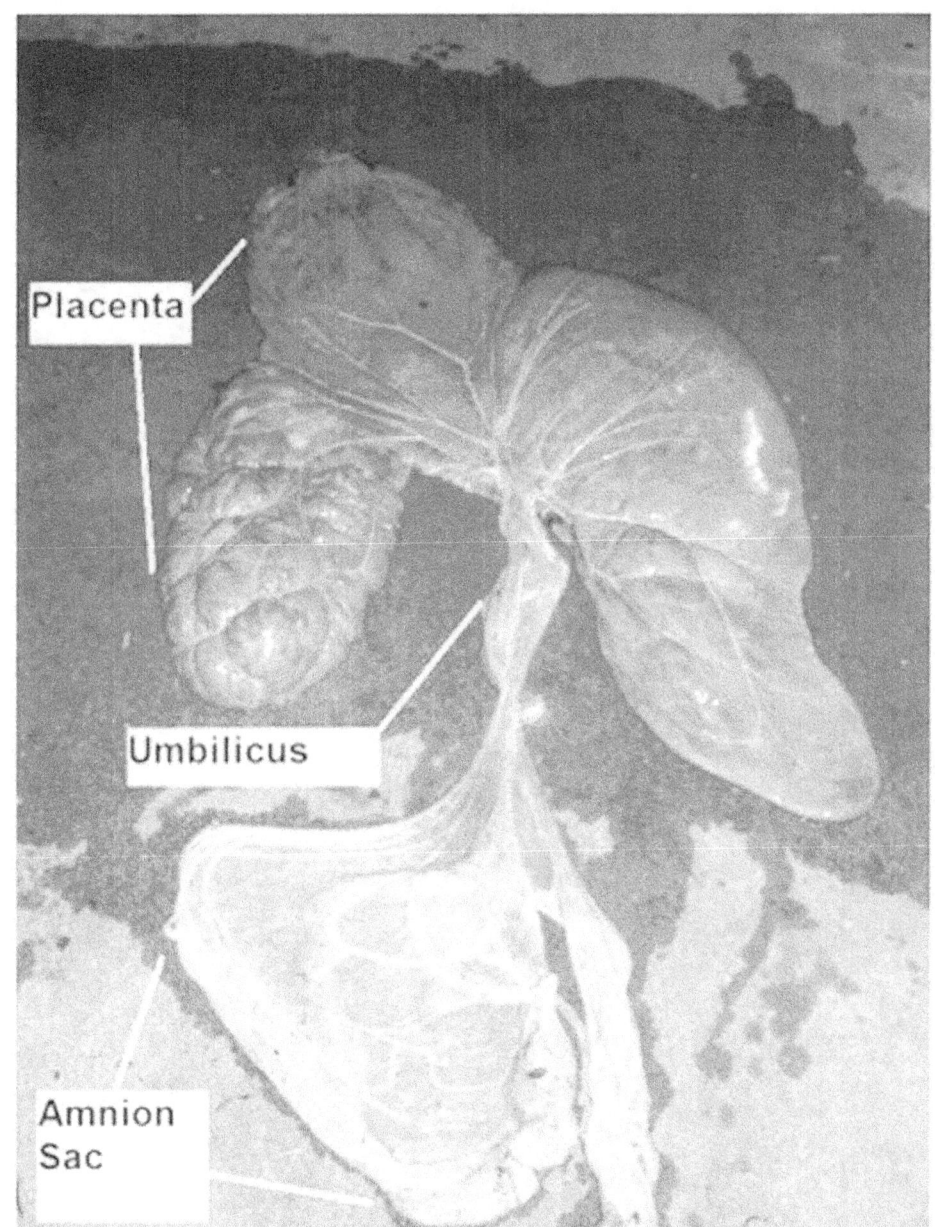

**Figure 4.9a:** *Complete passed placenta*

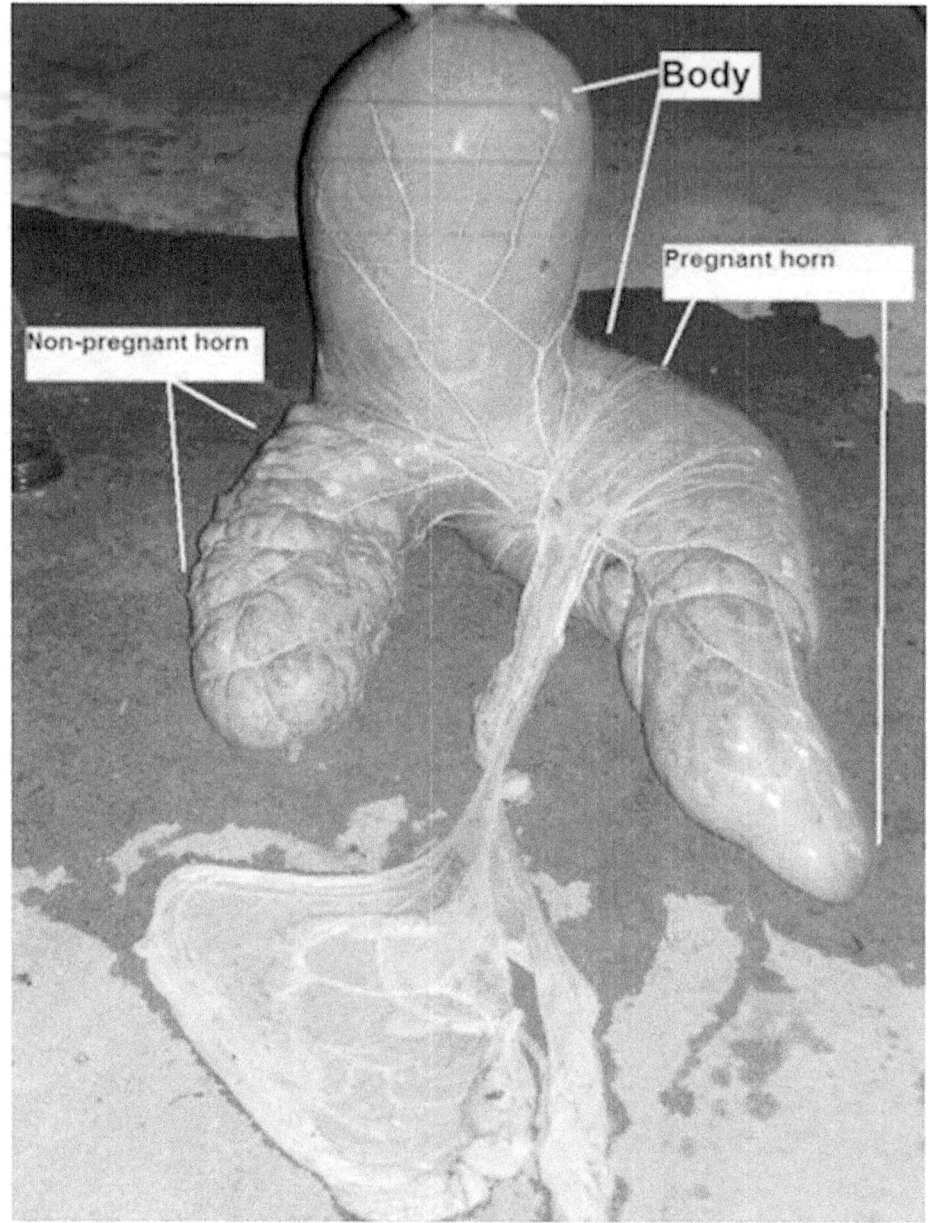

**Figure 4.9b:** *Complete placenta filled with air to show size*

## Conclusion

Of course the information discussed in this chapter is not all-inclusive. There are other conditions related to pregnancy that need emergency care. For example, uterine torsion can happen if the uterus flips over inside the mare. The diagnosis is made based on the history, physical exam, and careful rectal palpation by the vet. The point is that if something is out of the ordinary on your exam, you can discuss this with your vet and determine if the situation is an emergency. Never treat the horse with medications that will mask pain unless directed to by your vet.

Now that the mare has foaled, you have a new member in the family. In the next chapter we will explore problems that can arise in the newborn foal. These are termed neonatal emergencies.

# Neonatal Emergencies - The Newborn Foal

CHAPTER

## The First 24 Hours

Take a moment after the foal is born to let the mare clean the foal and allow the normal bonding to occur. Too much commotion and talking can agitate the mare, so if a lot of people are present at the time of delivery, make sure that the mare is not getting distressed. If there is a rejection by the mare to the foal you will have some major hurdles to overcome! Most mares are comfortable with their usual handlers, so one or two people outside the stall at a time is fine. Be sure to dip the foal's navel after cord separation. (See Chapter 2)

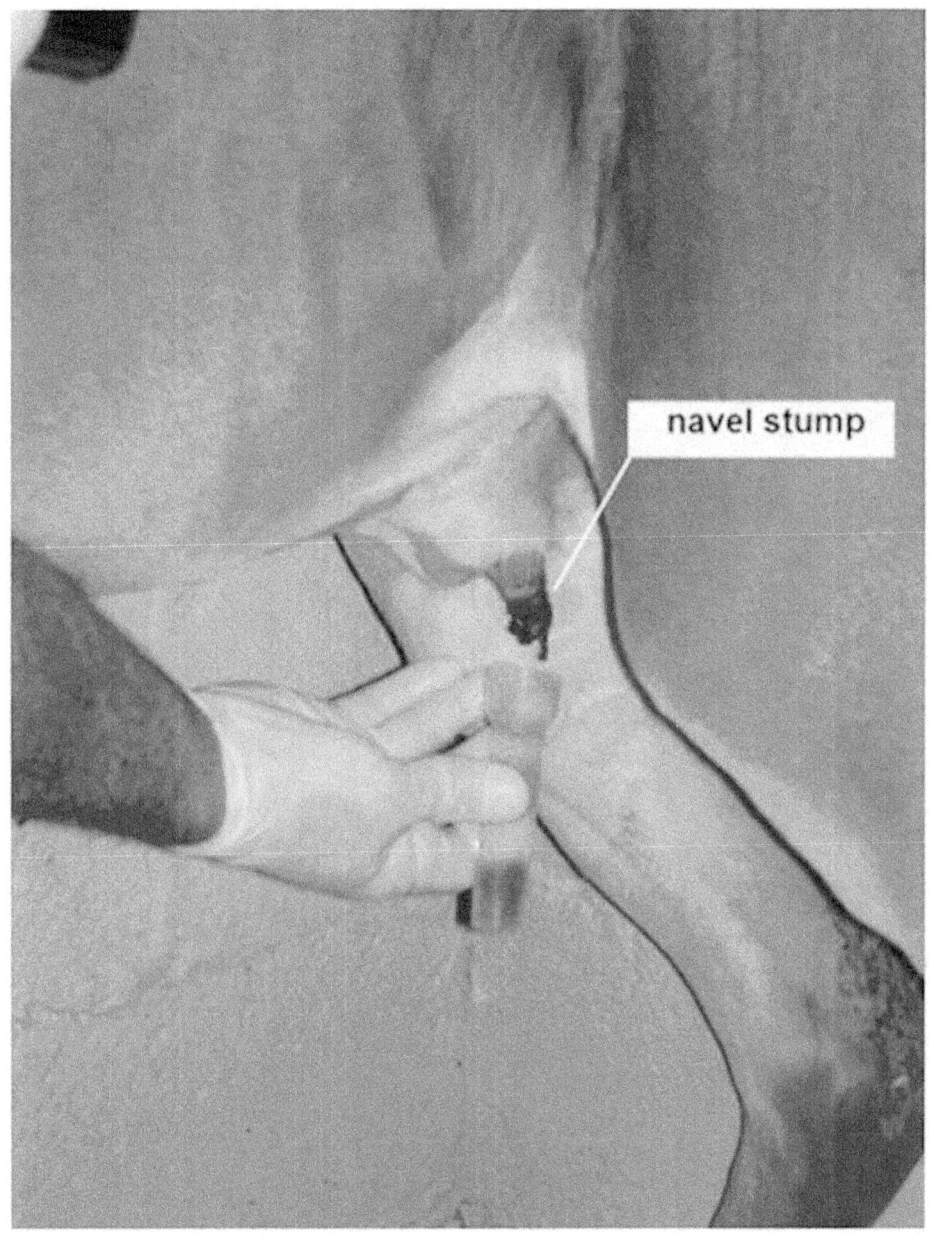

**Figure 5.1a:** *Naval stump*

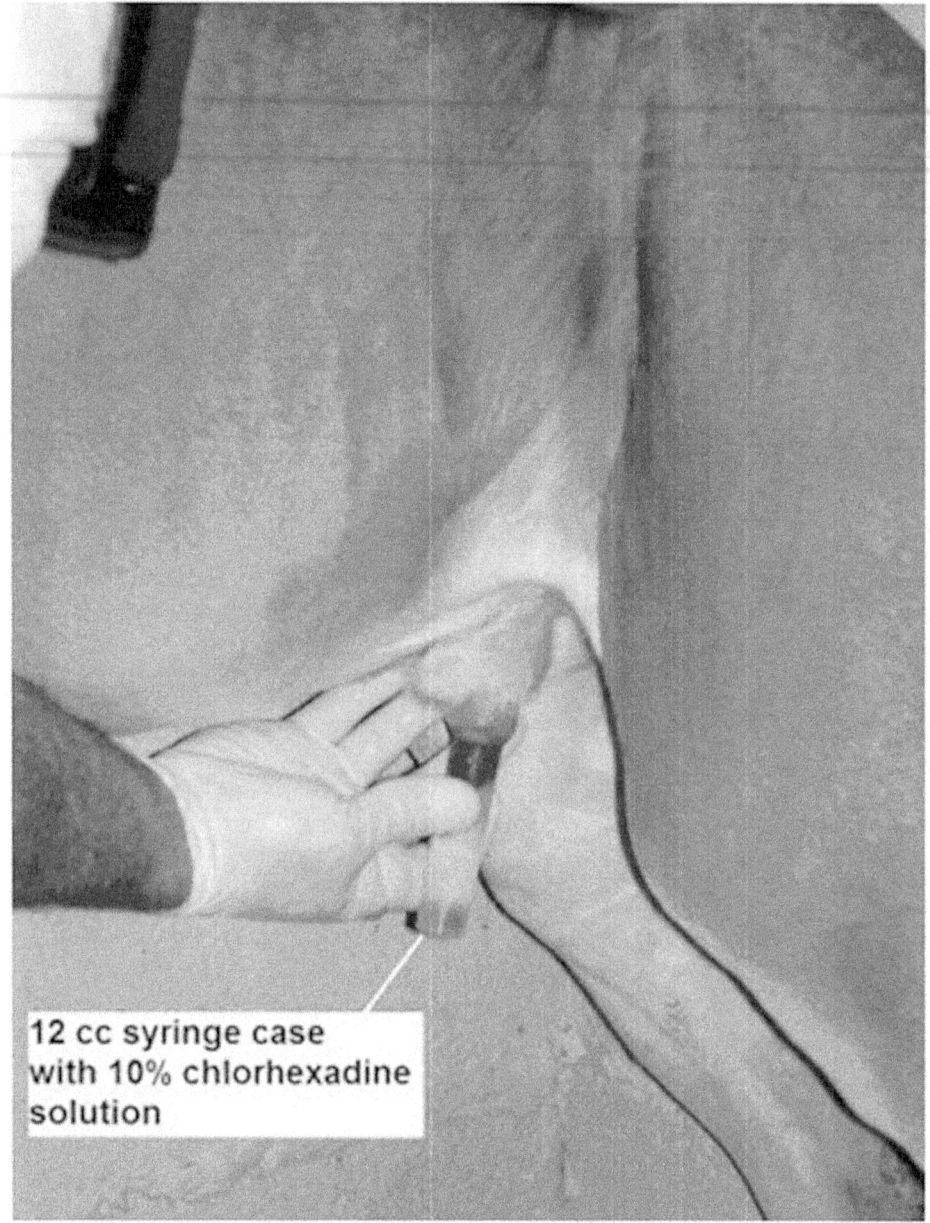

**Figure 5.1b:** *Application of naval dip*

From the moment the foal is born, there is a time frame of events that need to occur. First, the foal should stand in one hour. Several unsuccessful attempts may happen, but eventually they will get the hang of it! Next, the foal will nuzzle the mare looking for the udder. It is normal for the foal to take up to an hour to find the right spot. If you want to assist, we find that the most helpful way is to have an assistant stand on the opposite side while one stands behind the foal. A small amount of milk may be expressed from the teat towards the foal's nose. Sometimes we will place a few drops on a clean finger and entice the foal to the teat that way. It is imperative to let the foal find the teat on their own terms, as any forcing will cause the foal to become fatigued and want to lie down.

The foal should be nursing normally in the first 2-3 hours. It is imperative that the foal receive the mare colostrum (first thick honey-like milk) in the first 2-8 hours from birth. If the foal misses this opportunity, there is a risk that the foal's gut lining will close down and not receive the antibodies in the colostrum that offer protection from bacteria and viruses. In other words, there is a window of eight hours that the foal must nurse enough colostrum. If outside this window, the foal's gut will actually close and not allow absorption of the colostral antibodies.

Make sure to test the foal's blood around 18-24 hours to ensure adequate transfer of colostral antibodies. This is termed an IgG test and is commonly performed by your vet during the mare/foal check. Having a low transfer can subject the foal to a wide variety of diseases and infections. Plasma can be given if there is sufficient risk and the foal has had low to no transfer. However, there are risks associated with plasma treatment as well, so preventing the problem from the onset is obviously the best treatment. Being prepared with backup colostrum is also beneficial if the mare has inadequate or poor colostrum. Good colostrum can be banked in a freezer for a couple of years. The specific gravity of the colostrum can be measured to determine its antibody concentration. If frozen colostrum is needed, do not thaw in a microwave! This will damage the antibodies. Instead, use a warm water bath and then feed the foal with a bottle, or allow the vet to tube feed the foal.

## Mare/Foal exam

This exam is usually done by your veterinarian within the first 24 hours of birth. The exam consists of evaluating the mare for birthing injuries, udder quality, and placenta passage. Remember to save the placenta in a bucket or plastic bag. A routine physical exam of the mare is done as well to assess heart and respiratory rates and mucous membrane color.

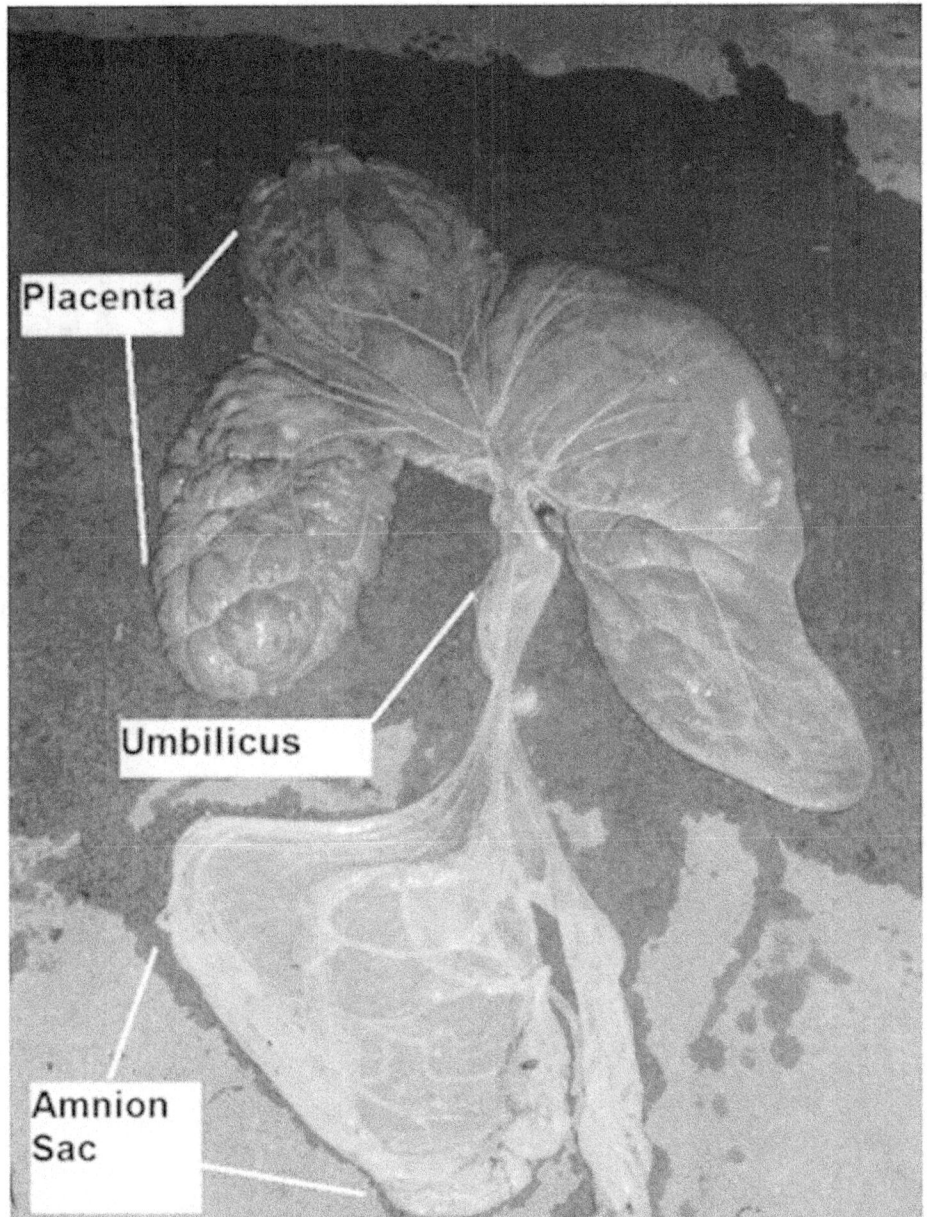

**Figure 5.2:** *Complete passed placenta*

The foal is also examined by assessing heart and respiration, temperature, stool and urination, navel cord, eyes, mouth (palate), possible hernias, and any limb abnormalities. Early detection is the key to treatment. Additionally, as mentioned previously, an IgG test is performed, especially if there is any concern that the foal was or is not nursing well, or if the mare's milk supply seems insufficient.

On occasion, the foal may have a meconium impaction. The meconium is the first stool produced by the foal. It can range in color from yellow-orange to brownish-black. An enema (Fleet™) can be administered if the foal is showing signs of constipation. An indication of constipation is when the foal raises his tail several times and strains with no result. If you are not experienced with administering an enema, discuss it with your vet or someone who has done it before. The tissue inside the rectum can easily be damaged, so being gentle and quick with the enema, as well as having the foal restrained properly for the procedure is essential. The meconium should be passed within the first 24 hours. When restraining the neonatal foal be sure to avoid trauma to the fragile rib cage. Using one arm around the front of the chest and one behind the back legs is usually sufficient.

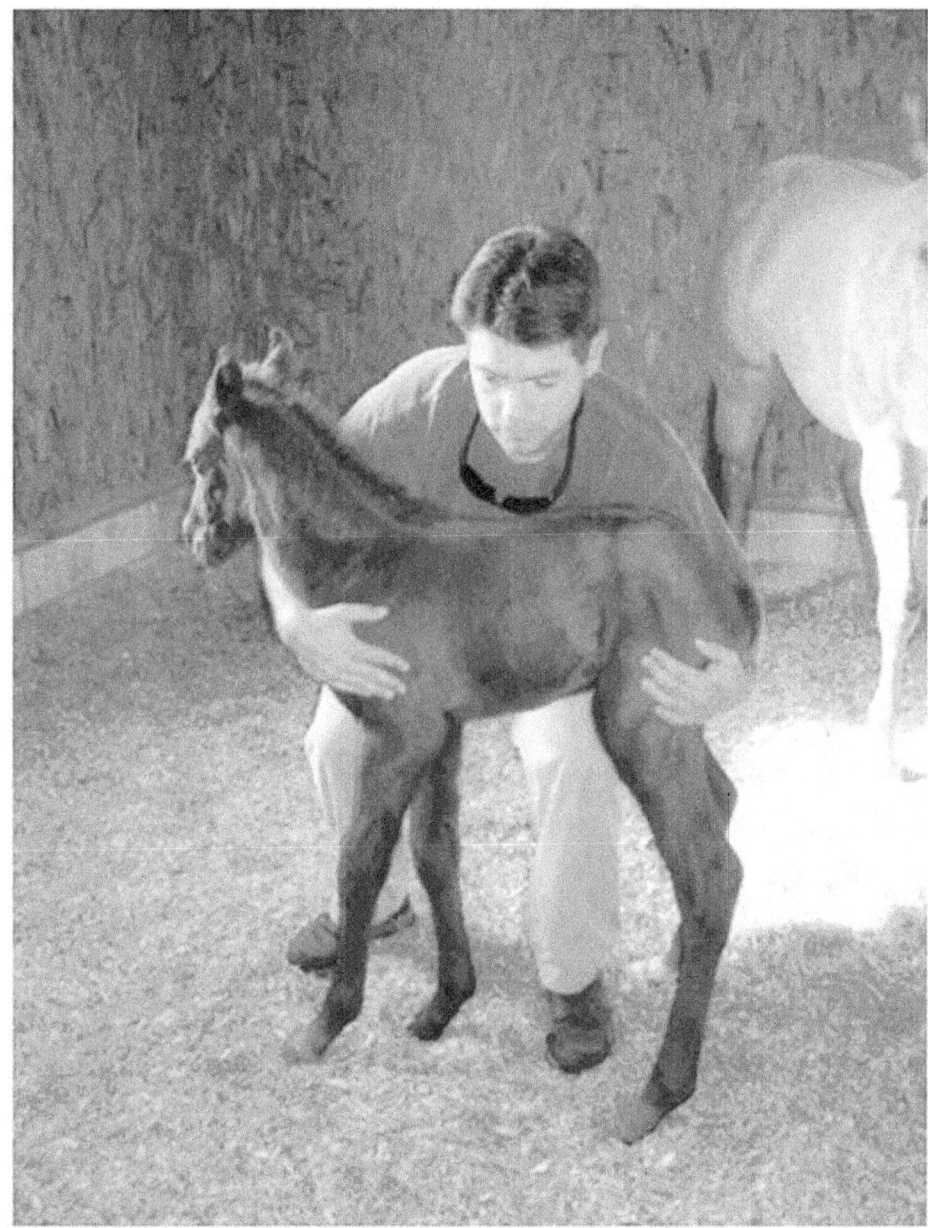

**Figure 5.3a:** *Proper restraint of a neonatal foal*

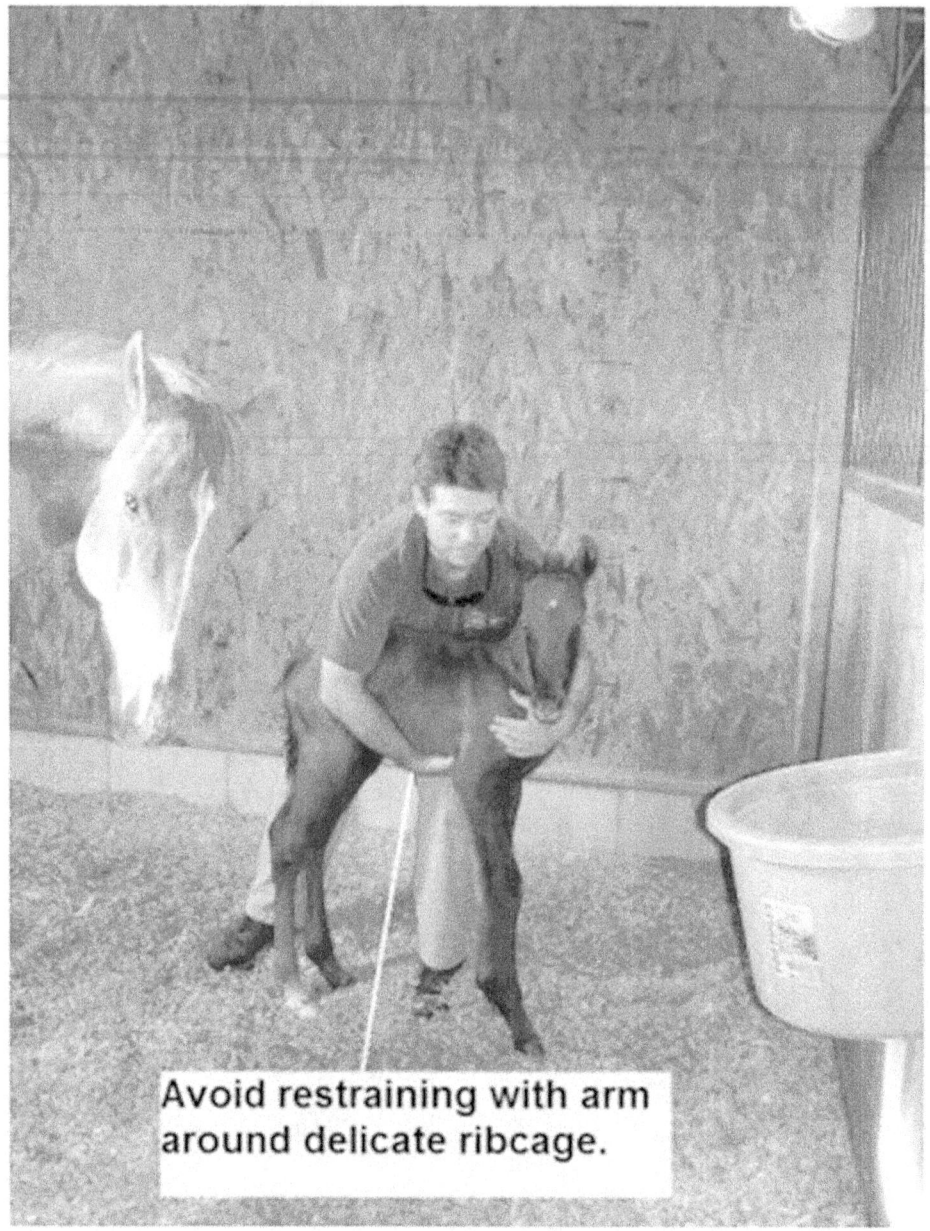

**Figure 5.3b:** *Avoid restraining a neonatal foal around the ribcage*

# Environment

Having the cleanest environment for foaling is quite helpful to avoid unnecessary infections. The foal is born without any antibodies to protect against certain diseases. Washing the mare prior to foaling can help to eliminate a lot of potential bacteria with which the foal could come into contact. Washing the udder and armpits is a good idea since the foal will be mouthing these areas when first trying to nurse. Straw bedding is also recommended since it is cleaner and less dusty than shavings. If the mare will be kept in a corral or fenced area, be sure that the lower margins of the fence are such that a small foal could not pass under. Such an event could separate the mare and foal thus causing the mare to risk severe injury to get back to her foal or vice versa!

# Normal vs. Abnormal

There are complete textbooks devoted to neonatal medicine. Our goal in this book is to allow you to make the determination of what is an emergency, not to touch on every aspect of foal medicine. If you know the normal parameters and find a problem, you can inform your vet of the situation and give vital information early that could thwart a huge problem later. Here are some guidelines for normal parameters.

## Normal Parameters

**Urination**: First at 12 hrs

**Defecation**: Within 12-24hrs. Any constant straining is abnormal.

**Appetite**: Must nurse adequately by 3-4 hours old. Any problem with suckling, swallowing, or milk supply should be addressed before the foal is older than 4-5 hours.

**Heart rate**: 90-120 bpm

**Respiration rate**: 40 bpm

**Temperature**: 100-101.5F. Temperature may be affected by outdoor temperature. Bring the foal indoors and take the reading when the foal is resting.

**Activity level**: Usually alternates between nursing 3-4 times per hour, sleeping, and exploration in the first 24hrs. Sleeping a lot, sluggishness, or wobbliness are signs that something is wrong.

## Neonatal Problems

- Prematurity
- Neonatal Maladjustment Syndrome
- Sepsis
- Colic/diarrhea
- Limb deformities
- Umbilical issues
- Mare Rejection
- Neonatal isoerythrolysis

## Prematurity

Prematurity is defined as foals born before 320 days gestation. However, the normal gestation lengths of individual mares and breeds can vary. In other words, if a mare normally carries a foal 365 days, then delivering at 335 days may be premature for that particular pregnancy. Therefore, you will have to rely on certain physical characteristics the foals will have if the foal is indeed premature. The characteristics are as follows:

- Short silky/velvety haircoat.
- Domed or prominent bulging forehead
- Weakened, lax tendons. Usually best seen in the fetlocks.
- Muscle weakness. Taking an abnormally long time to stand.

- Small size, low birth weight.
- Folded or floppy ears.
- Poor suckle response

Premature foals have premature body systems. The lungs and gut do not function at the normal capacity. In most cases, these foals should be admitted to an appropriate facility that has on site lab and life support capability. Until the foal can be examined by your vet and transported to a hospital if so desired, provide the best supportive care you can. You can milk the mare's colostrum and bottle feed the foal if possible. If the foal does not suckle, then the vet can give the colostrum via a stomach tube feeding. Never force the feeding with a bottle. The foal may inadvertently breathe in the fluid, thus causing an aspiration into the lungs which could lead to pneumonia. Keep the foal wrapped in blankets to conserve as much body heat as possible. If the foal is lying flat on their side, turn the foal every half hour or so to prevent any sores. Also, protect the foals eyes from the bedding by using a towel and/or triple antibiotic eye ointment in the eyes. The prognosis for premature foals is guarded even with the best medical care.

## Neonatal Maladjustment Syndrome

Neonatal Maladjustment Syndrome (NMS) is known also as dummy foal or barking foal syndrome. In textbooks, it is referred to as Hypoxic Ischemic Encephalopathy and Peripartum Asphyxia. As the textbook names imply, this condition is brought on as a result of oxygen deprivation to the foal at the time of delivery. This condition can occur in a normal term pregnancy that showed no outward sign of complications at delivery. Some foals may actually appear normal for several hours before showing any clinical signs.

Several factors are thought to play a role in the development of this syndrome. Early detachment of the umbilical cord or placenta during delivery or various diseases of the placenta are believed to contribute to the cause. For the most part diligent supportive care is all that is needed to help the foals through this problem. In worst case scenarios, some foals will need anticonvulsant medications and/or anti-inflammatory medications to control seizures and reduce inflammation in affected body organs. In foals that are severely compromised, antibiotics are usually administered to prevent secondary infections.

If the foal cannot nurse, a nasogastric feeding tube can be placed to provide essential nutrition. To prevent dehydration and low blood sugar, some foals require intravenous fluid therapy. The lack of oxygen can affect the brain, gut, kidneys, heart and lungs. Some foals may show signs with all or some of the body systems, so here is what to look for:

**Brain** - Aimless wandering and disorientation. Foals may appear blind and lose their suckle reflex. Some foals may exhibit a head tilt. Some foals may be overly sensitive to outside stimuli such as noises, light, and touch. In worst cases, foals may have seizures and muscle tremors or coma. During seizures, there may be awkward vocalizations that resemble dog barking. Foals that have neurological signs associated with NMS can have a full recovery. However, if the foal has fixed, dilated pupils unresponsive to light from brain damage, the prognosis for survival is poor.

**Kidney** - Foals may have increased frequency or lack of urination.

**Gut** - Foals may have outward signs associated with colic. There may be diarrhea and bloating in the belly.

**Lungs** - Respiratory distress, increased respiratory rate, or difficulty breathing.

**Heart** - An increase heart rate, heart murmurs, abnormal rhythm, and low blood pressure (check pulses).

Overall, NMS is not necessarily a death sentence. Affected foals can be saved with diligent supportive care. Ensure the foal gets adequate nutrition and hydration, protect the foal from bodily harm associated with seizures, and institute medical therapy if needed in severe cases. Most foals with NMS have recovered and developed into normal healthy horses without long term side effects.

## Sepsis

Sepsis is defined as having the presence of bacteria and/or their associated toxins in the bloodstream and tissues. Obviously a serious condition, septic foals can be in immediate life threatening danger. Foals usually become septic as a result of weakened bodily defenses. For instance, a foal that has not received adequate colostrum is at risk of infectious diseases and sepsis more than a foal who had received adequate colostrum. Also, premature foals often succumb to sepsis due to their weakened body defense systems.

A septic scoring system has been developed that uses various blood tests and physical exam findings to assign a numerical value to a sick foal. This score helps the vet to determine if a foal is at a higher risk of sepsis, without actually culturing the blood. Behavioral cues that can tip you off to a septic foal can be as simple as the cessation of nursing or a large distended udder in the mare. A weak or lame foal with or without an increased temperature is also a warning sign. Septic foals often have diarrhea as well. Obviously, if you are in tune to the normal parameters of a healthy foal, and find abnormalities, call your vet to discuss the problem as soon as possible. Treating a septic foal early at the onset of trouble is vital for a successful outcome.

## Colic/Diarrhea

Colic can be defined as moderate to severe pain emanating from the abdomen. Foals show similar signs of colic as adults such as rolling and looking at their sides. In horses, the most common cause of colic is due to a problem with the bowel. In foals, there are a couple common causes of colic. Meconium impactions occur when the meconium, or first stool, becomes impacted in the colon. Foals with meconium impactions will stop nursing, strain frequently with no result, show signs of colic pain, and may have abdominal distention. Most impactions resolve with an enema; however, some stubborn impactions may require specialized enemas that are medicated and given under light sedation or anesthesia. Rarely surgery may be required.

Another cause for colic is enteritis (inflammation of the bowel). Enteritis usually occurs from bacterial and/or viral infections. The foals will have a decreased or absent appetite and will often show rapid signs of dehydration. Symptoms of dehydration include increased heart and respiration rate, dry mucous membranes, and prolonged skin tenting. Chapter one provided information on assessing hydration using skin tenting. Instead of tenting the skin at the neck, use the skin just above the upper eyelid. Oftentimes, the eyes may look sunken as well. These foals require immediate intravenous fluid therapy. A fever can sometimes accompany the enteritis. Diarrhea will also be present most times. Coupled with the fact that the foal is not nursing and losing further fluids from the diarrhea, the urgency for fluid therapy is justified.

Be sure to isolate any foal with diarrhea to avoid spreading the infection to other foals. The stall should be thoroughly disinfected with appropriate cleaners after the horses have been moved out. Place a foot bath of diluted bleach outside the stall if the foal is to be treated at your barn. A culture of the feces should be obtained to identify the infectious agent if possible. Serial culturing, or culturing daily for at least 5 days, should be done if your veterinarian suspects Salmonella.

Foals will most times have a foal-heat diarrhea. This occurs around the time the mare has her first heat cycle post-foaling. On average it will happen anywhere from day 5-12 post-foaling. The foals are still nursing and quite alert other than the loose stool. Within a few days or less the diarrhea stops as quick as it started. Unless the foal is showing other signs of sickness, such as not nursing, there is no need for any therapy. Some people choose to give a probiotic, which is fine.

## Foal pneumonias

Several agents both bacterial and viral can be responsible for foal pneumonia. These will be discussed in the respiratory chapter.

## Limb Deformities

Limb deformities are relatively common in the newborn foal. Fortunately, most are mild and many require no treatment, just patience. Foals may be born with contracted legs, lax or weak legs, or angular deformities (bent legs). During the mare/foal exam, your vet will evaluate the foal's legs.

In my experience, the most common deformity seen is lax or weak legs. This is mostly seen in the hind limbs at the fetlocks, but it can be seen in all four limbs. If the foal is able to stand and get around reasonably well to nurse, there is no treatment needed. The vast majority of these foals will start to strengthen their limbs in a few days up to a week or so with turnout and free exercise. If the limbs are weak enough so that the fetlock is touching the ground, then a therapeutic glue-on shoe can be used to provide support and more or less help the foot to stand flat on the ground.

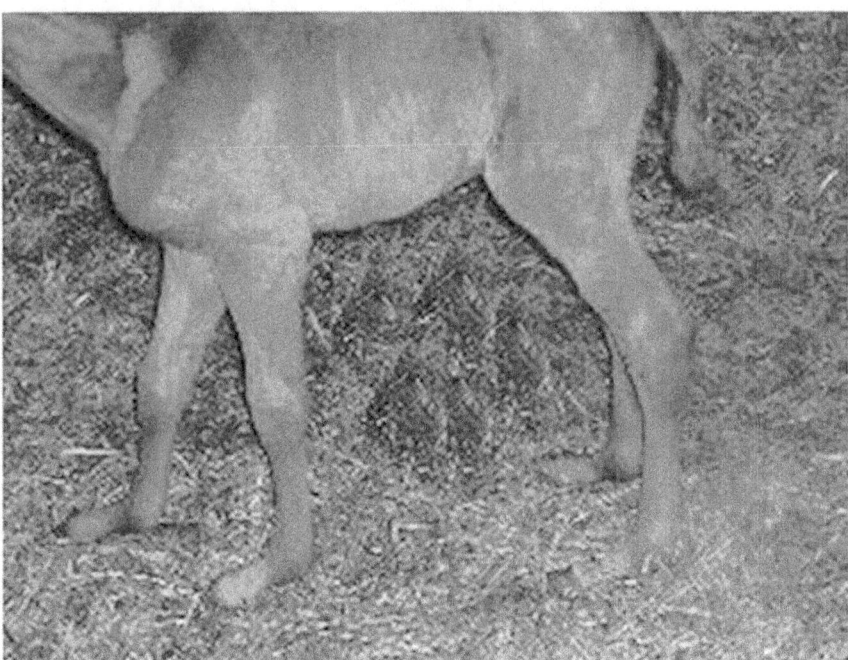

**Figure 5.4:** *Lax flexor tendons in newborn*

Another method is to tape a tongue depressor or two to the sole of the foot so that the tongue depressor extends a couple inches past the heels, thus forcing the toe down. Bandaging and support wraps should be avoided in most cases. Due to the laxity of the legs, the bandages can cause uneven pressure on certain points of the leg leading to open wounds.

If the foal is contracted in the limb(s), you may see the foal walking on their toes and trembling at the knees (carpus). Early treatment with oxytetracycline intravenously for up to 3 days helps many foals relax and allow the tendons to stretch.

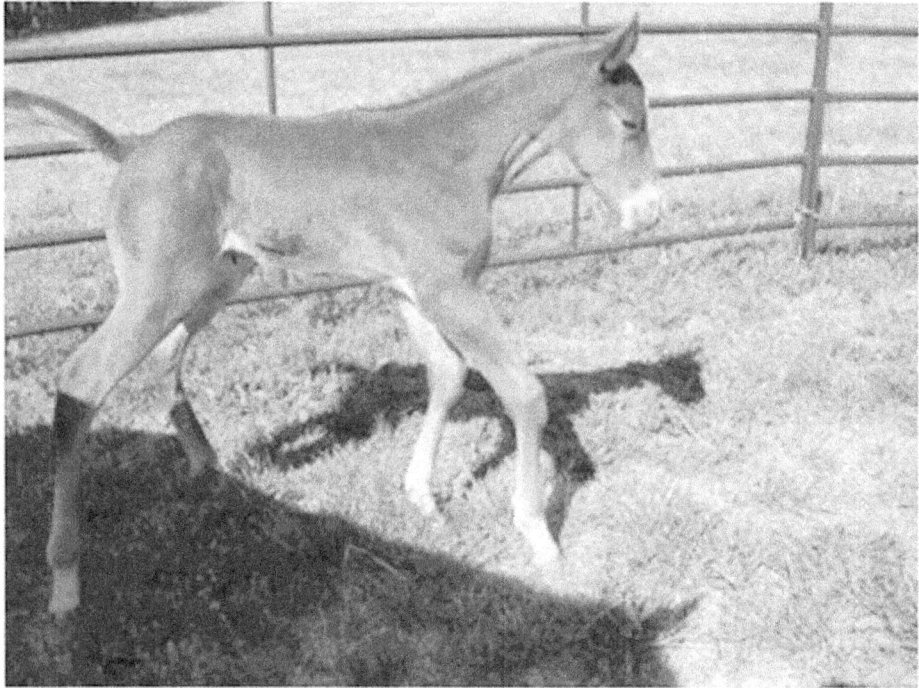

**Figure 5.4:** *Neonate foal with contracted carpus (knees)*

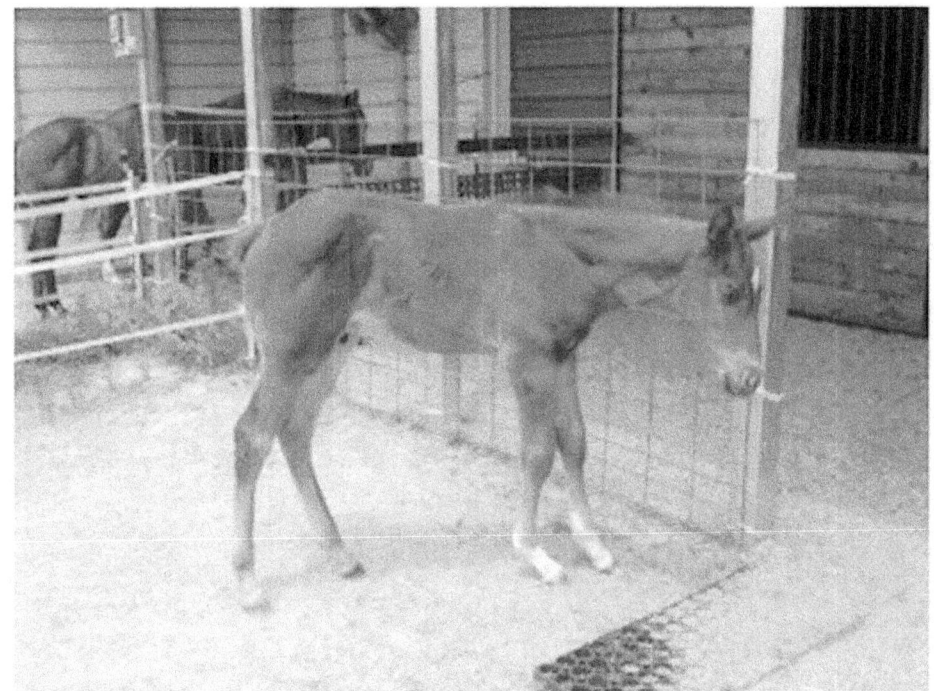

**Figure 5.4b:** *Same foal at 2 months*

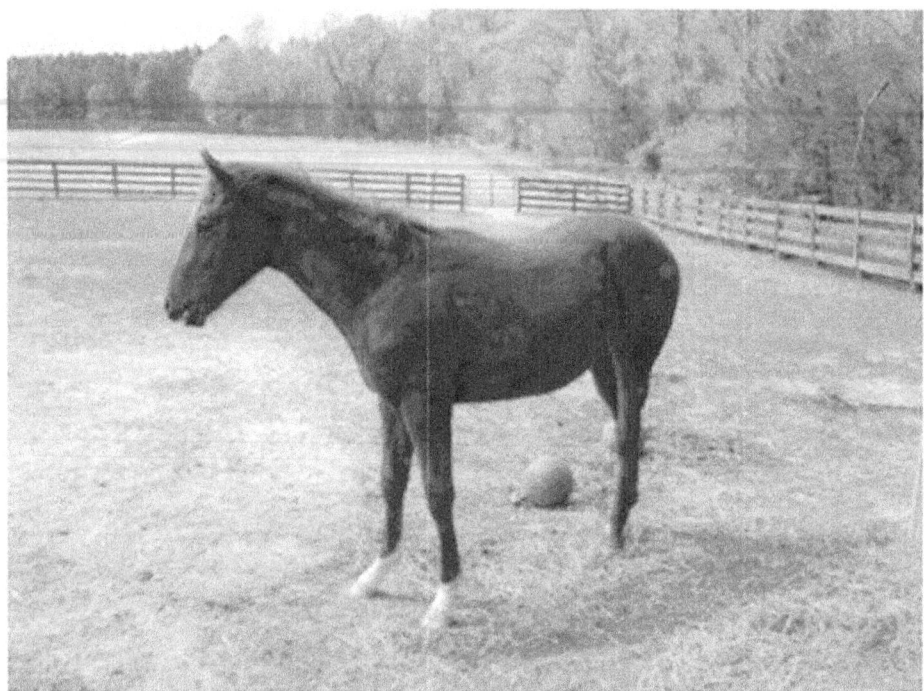

**Figure 5.4c:** *Same foal as a yearling*

Oxytetracycline is an antibiotic; however, it has a property that causes calcium to be bound in the body which in turn causes muscles to relax. Since the tendons are connected to muscles at one end this therapy often is effective at correcting contracted tendons. Most foals should be lightly sedated to receive the oxytetracycline. During this nap time you can help the vet by massaging the legs and stretching the contracted tendons. Some vets believe these foals should be kept in a stall since any exercise may have a negative effect by tensing up the muscles and not allowing the tendons to relax. Remember in mild cases there is usually no need to treat medically. These foals can do well by regular massaging and stretching while they are lying down.

Angular deformities are determined by evaluating the foal looking from the front or from behind. More often, the angle is deviated from the foreleg past the knee (carpus) or the thigh past the hock. Again, most of these foals will recover spontaneously, therefore patience is important. I do not suggest a surgical approach until the foal is at least 6-8 weeks old or older for limbs that do not straighten spontaneously. The surgical treatment is aimed at stimulating bone growth or lengthening of the limb on one side just above the joint that is bent.

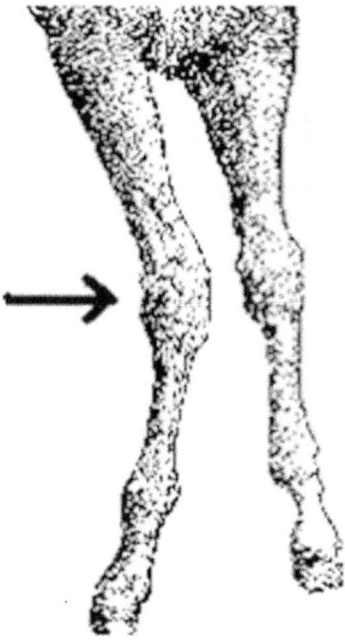

**Figure 5.5:** *A windswept foal-carpus valgus*

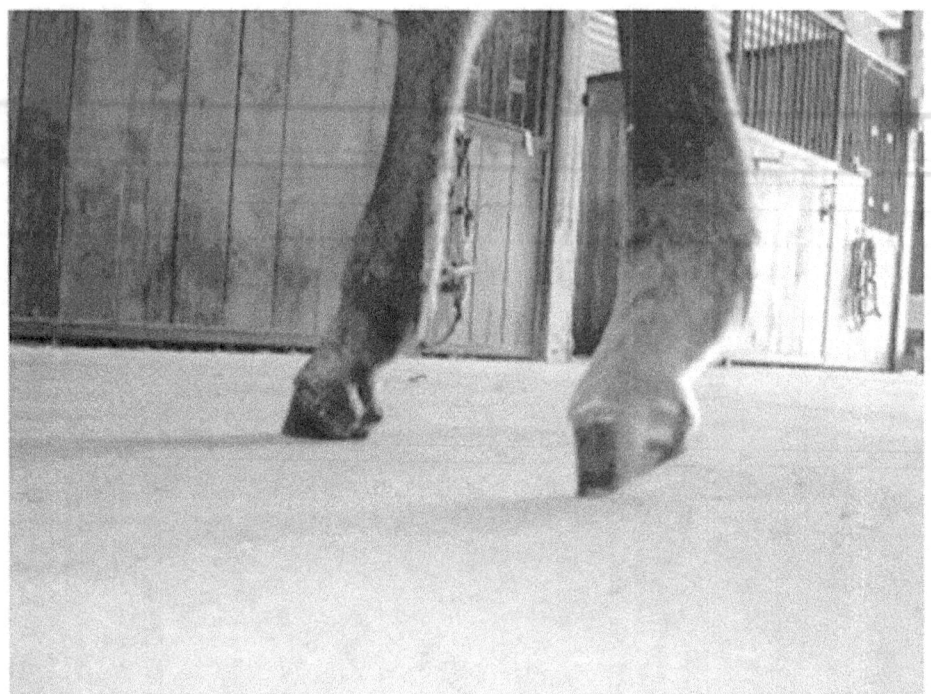

**Figure 5.6:** *Contracted tendon of left fore leg*

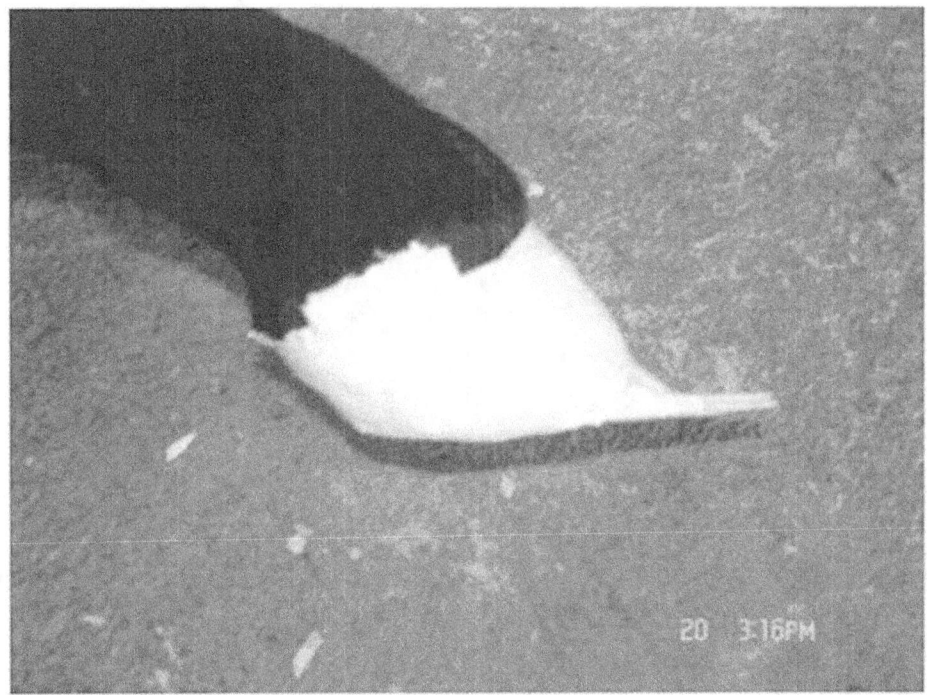

**Figure 5.7:** *Tongue depressors taped to contracted leg*

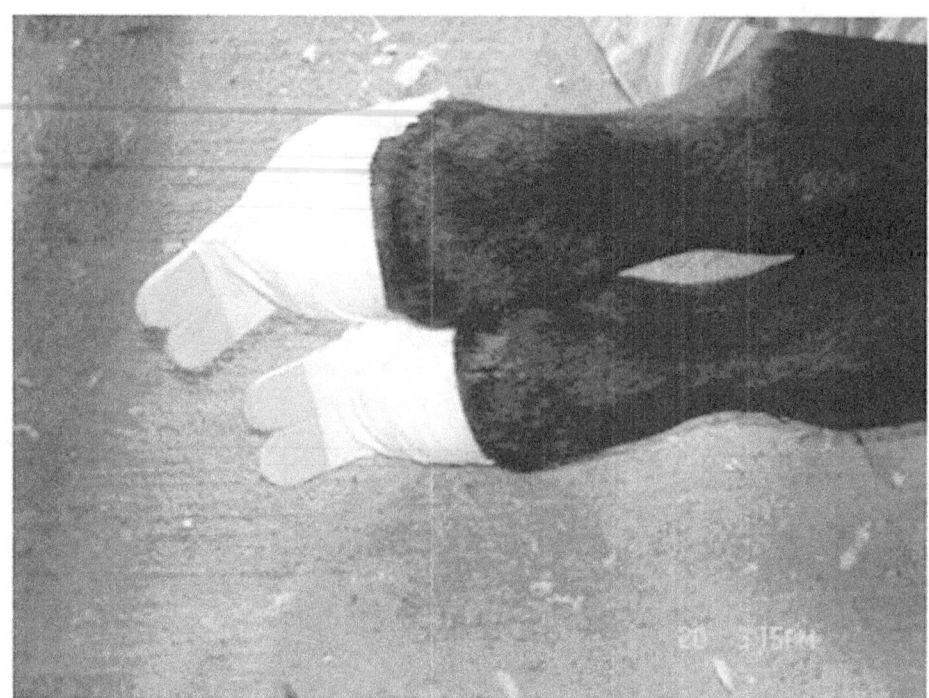

**Figure 5.8:** *Tongue depressors taped to extend toes*

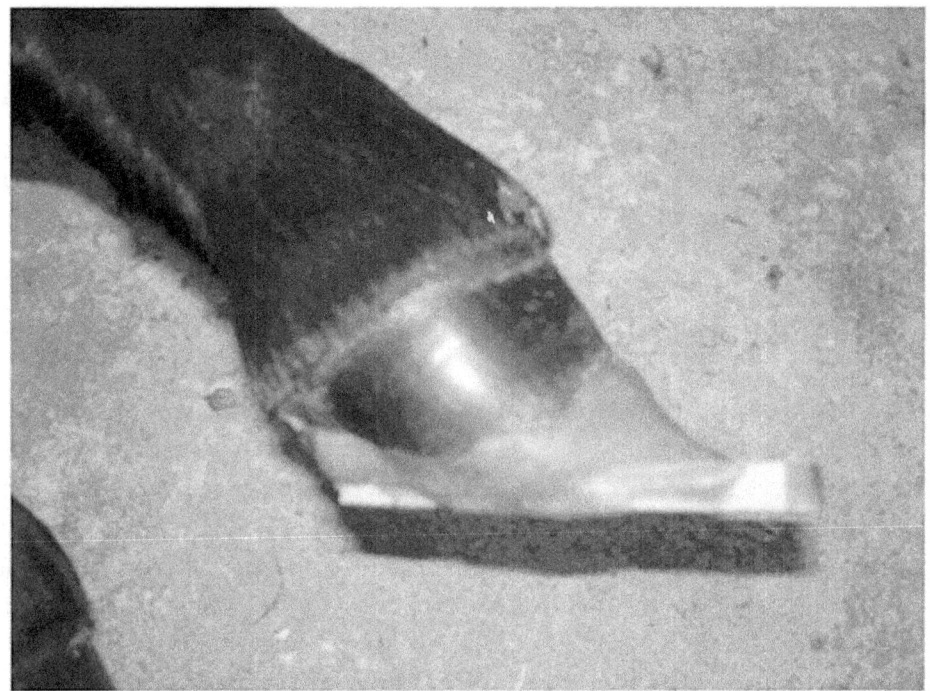

**Figure 5.9:** *Wooden extension glued to foot to extend toe and promote stretching*

## Umbilical Diseases

The umbilicus or navel can be a route for bacteria to enter the foal's body in early life. That is why it is recommended to disinfect the navel early by dipping. In any event the navel or umbilicus can have complications. Look for any increase in size or drainage (clear or opaque). If there is swelling but it can be reduced easily without signs of fever or tenderness, the foal may have a hernia. This is not life threatening, but should be addressed if you can introduce more than a finger width into the hernia. Your vet should evaluate any drainage from the umbilicus.

Sometimes the urachus, which is essentially a tube that connects the bladder to the umbilical cord in utero, does not close at birth. This is termed a patent urachus. There will be urine dripping from the navel, which tends to stay wet. It can be treated medically by applying silver nitrate sticks to the stump to promote closure. If this is not successful, then surgery should be considered before potential infection occurs. If the foal's umbilicus becomes infected, an abscess could form that may deliver bacteria into the body and spread to other tissues such as the joints and growing bones. This is termed navel ill and requires immediate attention. Most foals exhibit a fever and will be lame on the affected limb(s).

## Mare Rejection

Of all the complications that can happen to your foal, this is a potential nightmare. The fledgling foal is doing their best to get that first meal and the mare shows no interest or may be overly protective and will not stand still for the foal to nurse. In worst cases, the mare may actually attack or kick the foal, which could be cause for immediate separation. Be aware that new mothers are more prone to this problem than seasoned mothers. This is one reason why it is important to keep noise levels and handlers down to a minimum during the birthing interval. Have other horses in the area removed so that the mare is not distracted.

Try to determine if the mare is being overly protective or really rejecting the foal. In some cases, the mare does not mind the foal's presence, but when the foal goes to nurse the mare may kick or move sideways. In this case, the mare's udder may be overly tender and sensitive. You can restrain the mare and try milking the colostrum into a bottle to feed the foal. Feed the foal close to the mare's udder to promote bonding.

If sedation is necessary consult with your vet as many sedatives can be excreted in the milk and transferred to the foal. Reinforce good behavior when the mare accepts the foal but try to avoid negative or painful correction when the mare misbehaves as this could teach the mare that the foal is a painful stimulus. You may feed the mare during the process to keep her mind on eating. A twitch can be applied to the mare if needed for the foal nurse. If done properly the twitch can release soothing endorphins to placate the mare while the foal nurses.

Remember this is only for short periods of time and should not reinforce the foal nursing as a negative occurrence.

When the mare does pass the placenta, leave it in the stall for a few hours. It is believed that the odor of the foal and the placenta are critical for normal bonding to occur. Gentle reinforcement goes a long way for the nervous mare. Be patient and keep in mind that most mares will accept their foal after you determine the cause for rejection.

## Neonatal Isoerythrolysis (NI)

Neonatal Isoerythrolysis is an uncommon, but sometimes fatal disease of the newborn foal. In simplest terms, the colostrum that is so essential for foal protection is the actual problem in this disease. Antibodies in the colostrum from the mare attack the foal's red blood cells causing them to rupture, leading to anemia. Affected foals will show signs of weakness and lethargy, high heart and respiratory rates, as well as jaundice, which is a yellow discoloration of eyes and mucous membranes. Definitive diagnosis is performed by testing the foal's blood, or performing a necropsy if the foal dies or is euthanized.

NI can be prevented in a couple ways. Blood typing the mare and stallion is helpful to determine if a cross-reaction may occur. High risk breeding should be avoided. Screening the mare's blood during the latter part of her pregnancy for antibodies to blood cells is another way to prevent NI. Any mare with a history of producing a foal with NI will be at a higher risk of producing another one in subsequent pregnancies. If the mare is already pregnant and confirmed to carry antibodies to the foal's red blood cells, the colostrum from that mare should be withheld from the foal. An alternate source of colostrum should be ready to administer to the foal. The mare's colostrum should be milked out thoroughly and discarded. It should be noted that mule pregnancies have a higher percentage of NI than horse pregnancies.

## Conclusion

This chapter covered some situations you may face during the first few hours and weeks of a foal's life. While not all-encompassing, this should give you an idea of the type of situations for which to be prepared when you are eagerly awaiting the birth of a foal.

The word colic can strike fear in the heart of even a seasoned horse owner. The next chapter will cover how to recognize colic and offer some guidance on ways to prevent it from happening. In addition to colic, other digestive problems will be reviewed.

# Digestive Emergencies  CHAPTER

## Colic

Without a doubt, every horse owner should be familiar with the word colic, and how it relates to horse emergencies. Colic is pain that emanates from the abdomen. With the horse, this pain is usually associated with a problem of the bowel. This pain can be mild to excruciating. These are some of the tell-tale signs:

- no appetite
- looking at sides
- pawing the ground
- walking in circles with head down
- laying down and rolling multiple times
- mouthing water but not drinking
- lip curling
- straining to defecate
- stretching out as if to urinate, and kicking up at the belly with hind limbs.

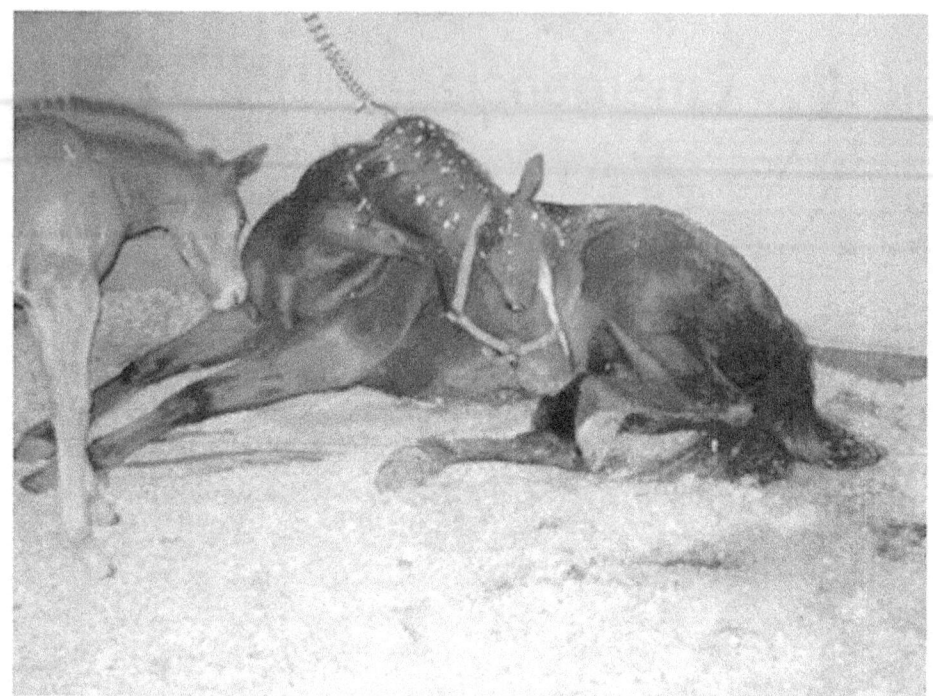

**Figure 6.1:** *Flank watching*

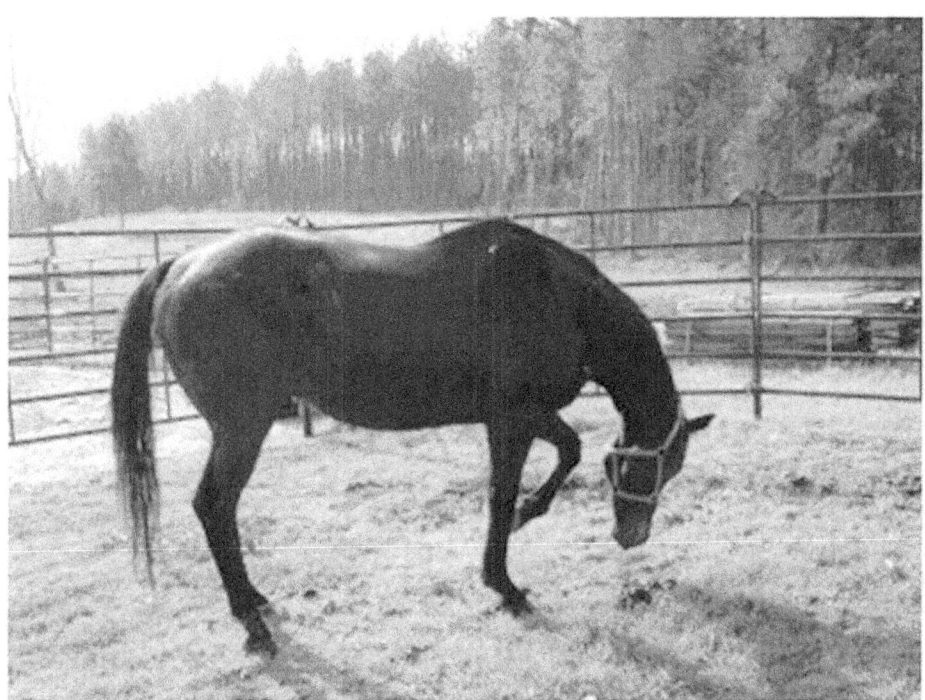

**Figure 6.2:** *Pawing at the ground*

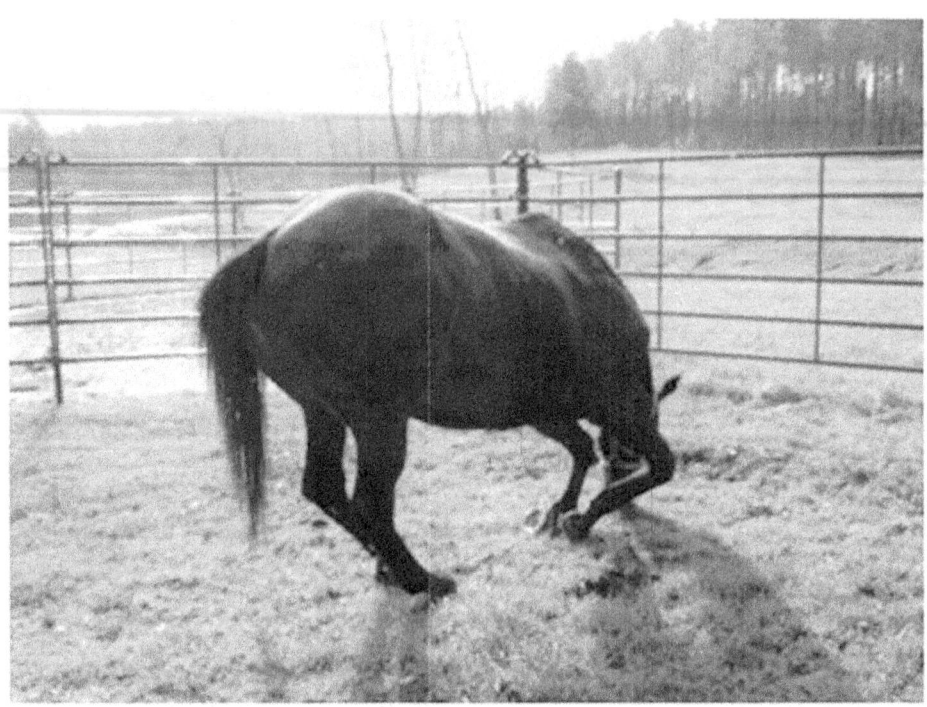

**Figure 6.3:** *Repeated attempts to lie down*

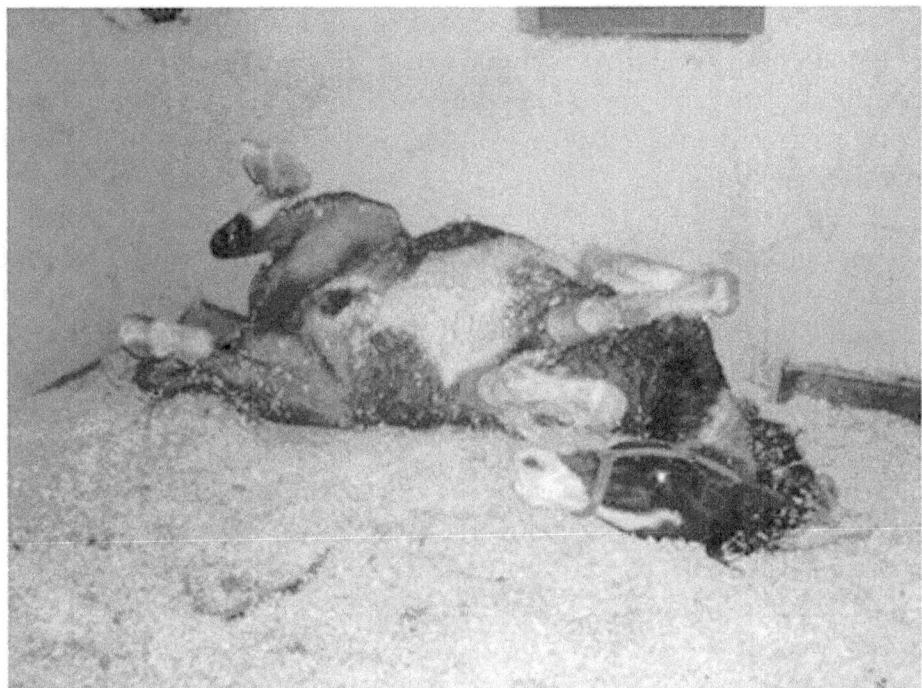

**Figure 6.4:** *Violent rolling*

Some horses exhibit only some of the signs while others may exhibit all. Bear in mind that one horse may not perceive pain as another horse would. So if two horses are suffering from the same type of colic, one may be stoic and not show outward signs of pain, while the other may be thrashing on the ground.

Colic is one of the most common of equine emergencies. It can also be said to be the number one killer of horses. It is an emergency that should not be taken lightly, as early treatment can be the key to a good outcome. Fortunately, most cases of colic are going to recover spontaneously. Still others may need medical therapy. Overall, a smaller percentage progress to life-saving colic surgery or euthanasia.

Rather than delve into the intricate processes that may cause colic in your horse, we will cover what can be done to prevent colic and what can be done in the event that your horse has developed colic. Horses possess a very large and lengthy intestinal tract that is always in motion since horses are naturally consuming most of the 24 hour day. Coupled with the fact that the bowels are quite mobile inside the large abdominal cavity, there is increased potential for trouble in horses more so than other large animals.

Preventing certain types of colic is easy if you follow a healthy, routine feeding program. Avoid sudden changes in your horse's feeding program. If a change is to be made, it should be done in a very gradual manner that slowly transitions the horse to the new diet by mixing new feed with old feed over a week or so.

Always have fresh water available as this is essential for normal bowel function. If the horse's water is dirty or frozen for example, then the decreased water intake may lead to impaction-type colic. Many colic cases can occur in the late fall or early winter as the normal water intake starts to decline.

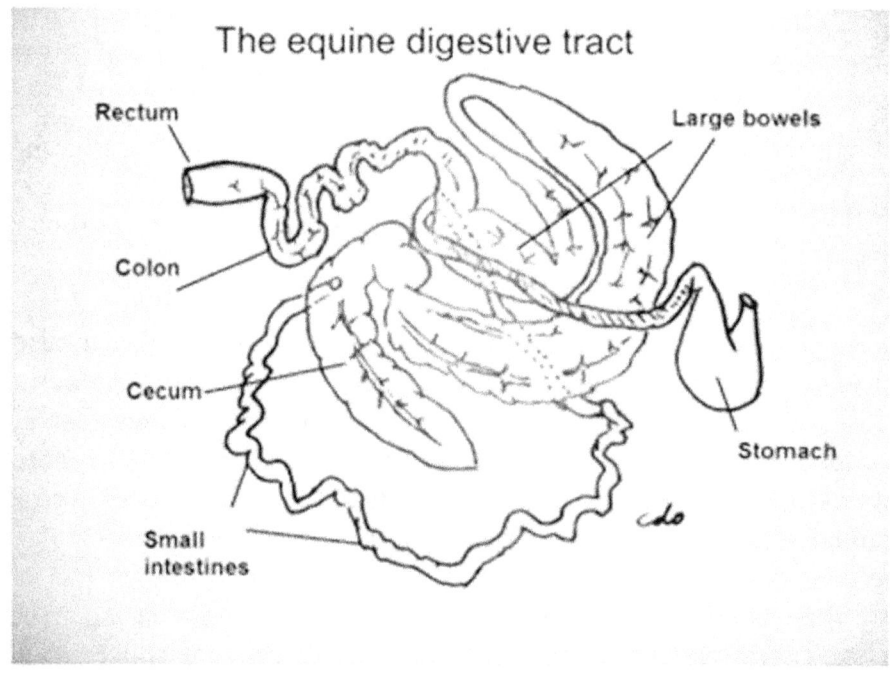

**Figure 6.5:** *Anatomy of Gastrointestinal Tract*

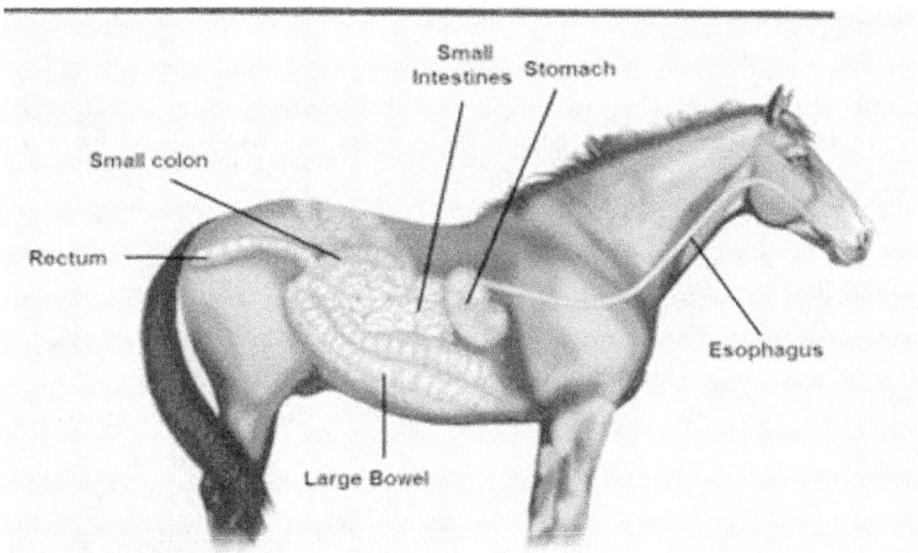

**Figure 6.5b:** *Equine GI Tract*

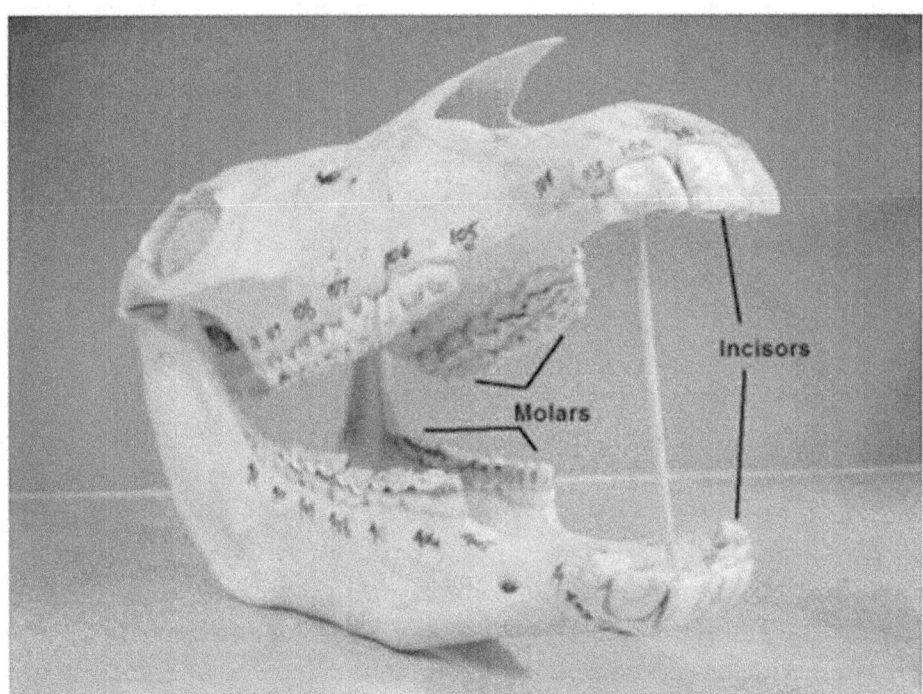

**Figure 6.5c:** *Equine skull exhibiting teeth*

## Colic Examination

Although it may be simple for some folks to know what ails their horse when colic is the culprit, other people (and horses) may have never experienced colic. It is important to familiarize yourself with the symptoms. Next, do a brief colic exam, if possible. I say *if possible* because in some cases the horse is in quite a bit of pain and will suddenly drop or turn without warning due to the pain. So be aware of the horses movement, and do not let yourself or others get hurt. I have been on calls when the handlers were so intent on keeping the horse up and walking that they had been injured when the horse fell into or even on them.

Try to incorporate a few of the techniques from Chapter 1 on doing a physical exam. As long as the horse is willing to stand still for a few moments, I will perform a gut sound evaluation first. Listen to all four quadrants for at least 30 seconds up to a minute. Next, assess the gum color and moistness. Next, do a skin tent to assess the horse's hydration. Next, take the horse's pulse under the jawline or listen to the heart with your stethoscope. Lastly, record a respiration rate. All this information will be valuable when you call your vet. Unless authorized by your vet, do not use any pain medication before they arrive. In a very few cases, I will ask my own clients to administer a small dose of pain medication before I can arrive. Very small doses are used so that pain is not masked before I perform my examination.

When your vet arrives, they will repeat most of your previous exam, and compare notes with you. In some cases, your vet may decide to perform a rectal exam to determine the cause of the colic. This exam should only be done by the vet! If performed by an inexperienced individual, the risk of causing an internal rectal tear could prove fatal to the horse. I will ask my clients for a thorough history on the horse's eating habits for the last 24-48 hours. The type of feed and hay is important to know as well as any drastic or sudden change in diet. Water intake, if measurable, is also helpful.

A thorough history can often lead me to a diagnosis. I will also ask the client if the horse is medically or surgically insured. If not insured, I will still ask if the client is willing financially to go forward with hospitalization and/or surgery if the horse's condition warrants. If there is any suspicion that the horse's condition would require hospitalization, then a call is made immediately to the referring hospital to discuss the horse's symptoms. Remember again, that it is best to treat aggressive in the earlier stages since waiting can cause rapid deterioration and possibly risk loss of the chance for a good outcome.

Further diagnostics can be performed on the horse that does not present with normal initial findings. These are best performed at the clinic or hospital since a laboratory setting is needed.

First, the horse's hydration status can be accurately assessed by performing a packed cell volume (PCV). A PCV is valuable information early in colic therapy since horses dehydrate quite rapidly during the colic episode. This test is done by obtaining a small drop of blood and drawing it into a very small glass tube to be centrifuged or spun down. All of the cells in the blood will be separated from the plasma or fluid part of blood. The tube is then set against a chart to determine the percentage of cells in the blood. This will give the clinician a way to determine how much fluid therapy, if any, is required to fix the deficit.

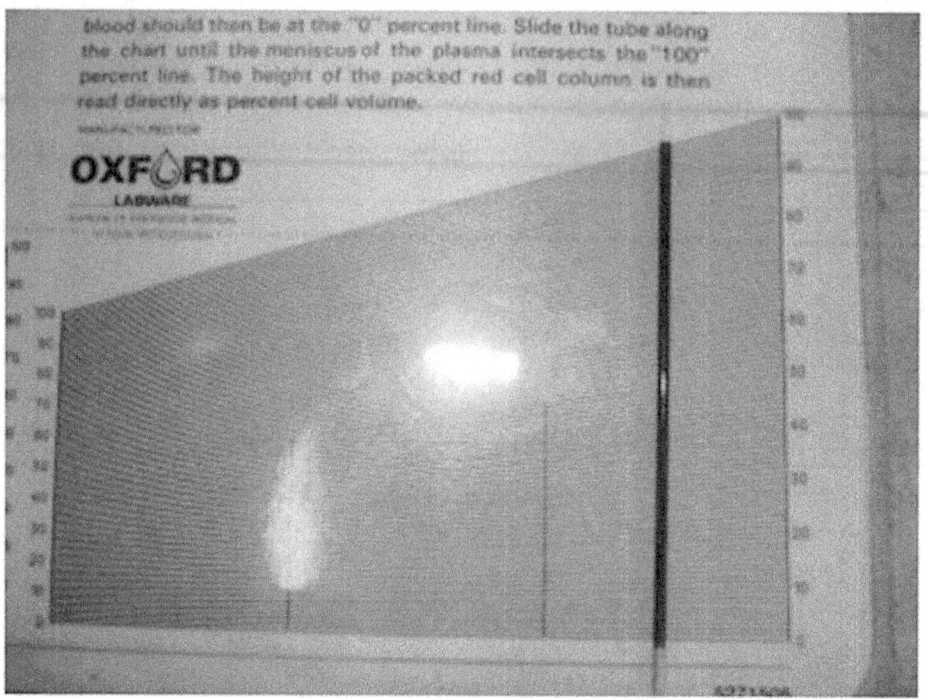

**Figure 6.6a:** *PCV blood tube before centrifuge*

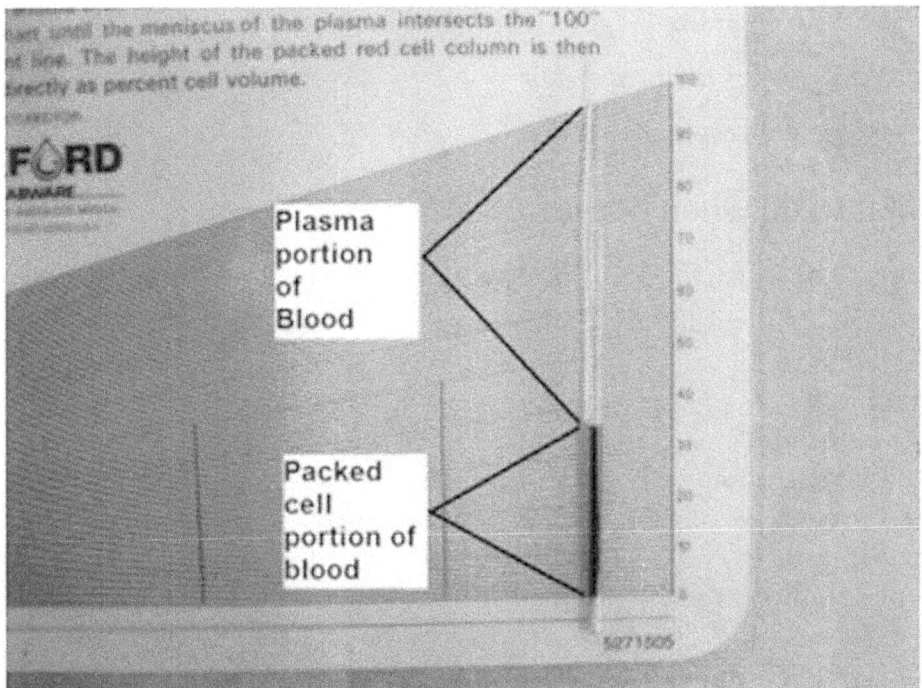

**Figure 6.6b:** *PCV blood tube after centrifuge*

Another useful diagnostic test is called abdominocentesis. This is a fancy way to say belly tap. Essentially a sterile area is prepped under the horse's abdomen, and a needle or cannula is inserted into the abdomen to obtain abdominal fluid for evaluation. Abdominal fluid bathes the internal organs. If there is disease, the fluid will have characteristic changes associated with color, cellular content and quantity, and the amount of fluid readily obtained. Some clinicians rely on the abdominal tap findings to know whether or not to go to surgery.

Another diagnostic test is an ultrasound of the horse's abdomen. Particular causes of colic can be determined in this exam and in some cases treated medically and resolved.

Here is a summary list of the evaluations to perform when attempting to diagnose colic:

- Gut sounds, all four quadrants

- Mucous membrane (gum) color and moistness
- Skin tent for hydration status
- Heart and respiratory rate

## What to do when horses colic

If you see that your horse is not interested in eating, without showing some of the typical colic signs as mentioned previously, take the horse's temperature first. A horse with a fever will oftentimes lose their appetite. These horses may or may not be colicky so proceed with the rest of your exam. Finish your physical exam by evaluating gut sounds, mucous membranes, heart and respiration rates, and skin tent. If there are subtle signs of pain such as lip curling, flank watching, and pawing the ground, try walking the horse for 15 to 30 minutes. It is always better to have the horse in an open area. The horse may have gas cramps and most times this will resolve the problem.

Be sure to call your vet to discuss your exam findings and set up a time frame so that if the horse is not resolving within the next hour he can be treated. If you have had a horse treated for colic or know someone who has, you may be familiar with some of the common treatment. Of course, the treatment plan between vets will vary, but it is common for horses to be administered a pain medication such as Flunixin (Banamine™) or Phenylbutasone along with a laxative given by nasogastric tube. Be aware that before anything is administered by nasogastric tube, the stomach of the horse should be refluxed or checked for fluid distention and relieved first.

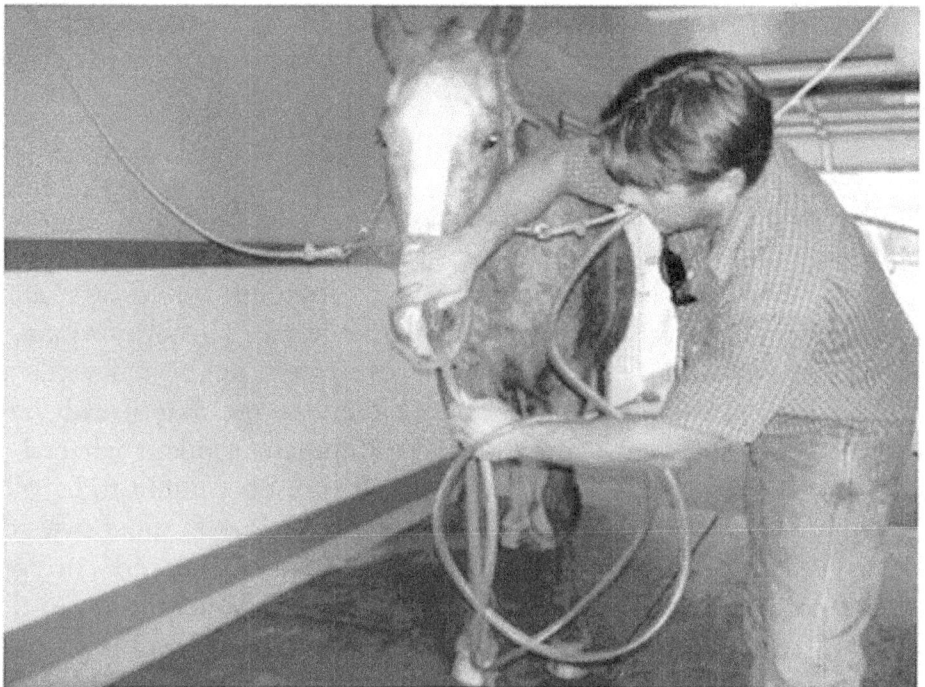

**Figure 6.7:** *Passing a nasogastric tube*

An interesting note is that horses are not capable of regurgitation or vomiting to relieve excess fluid or pressure in the stomach. In the event that a horse does have excessive stomach fluid build up, a nasogastric tube must be passed to remove the fluid. In some cases as much as five gallons can be siphoned off. These horses may have a heart rate of 80-90 beats per minute. If the excess fluid is not removed, the stomach can actually rupture from the pressure. This results in immediate shock and certain death.

Never administer a large laxative therapy orally to a horse. The horse will not readily take the treatment and could actually aspirate the treatment. This means instead of swallowing, the treatment could be inadvertently breathed into the lungs. I have treated horses that were given large amounts of mineral oil by their caretakers with a syringe orally. It was unfortunate to inform them that their horse now was dealing with aspiration pneumonia from the oil. Even if the colic resolved, the horse was now in jeopardy of life threatening pneumonia from the oil being aspirated into the lungs. I hope you can pass this on to anyone who feels that the horse should be given mineral oil orally first, then call the vet if there is no improvement!

Another point that I wanted to address is walking your horse during an episode of colic. It seems that the general belief of many caretakers is that if the horse were to lie down and roll, the guts would twist and all would be lost at that point! Not true. If the horse is in serious pain, and cannot stay on their feet despite being whipped on the tail while four people are screaming at the poor animal, then the gut may already have a twist or what I refer to as a torsion or entrapment. This is where I may lose some people. Please understand that it is not my intent to list all the ways a horse's gut can twist, but be aware that the gut in most cases does not really simply twist. In fact, the gut can become displaced, entrapped, torsed and even strangled by some fatty tumors. All of these can occur while the horse is standing. Consequently, if the horse was in one of these colic predicaments, lying down and rolling is not going to cause the gut to twist because the damage or twist is already done. If you can not keep the horse on his feet, try to consult with your vet to get some pain medication on board as soon as possible.

While on this subject, another common misconception is if the horse is passing stool, the colic is getting better. Not true. Realize that the last part of the bowel or the rectum can hold a good pile or two of stool. The colic problem may be further in front of the rectum and thus passing stool has no relevance early in the colic episode. If the horse seems to be recuperating and the pain improves over a 24 hour period, and then passes a few piles of stool; this is an excellent sign the problem is improving. Keep in mind that what a horse eats today will not show up in the manure for about three days.

## Causes of Colic

The good thing to know about colic is that most times the cause is not life threatening, and in many cases can resolve in a short period of time.

The following sections will cover some of the more common types and list a few of the least common.

## Impaction Colic

Impaction can occur in the equine intestinal tract when a bolus of feed material becomes lodged inside the intestines. There are a few areas inside the digestive tract where the bowel suddenly changes in size from a large diameter to a small diameter. Impactions are most likely to occur in these areas.

Initially, horses may not show any sign other than a loss of appetite or finicky eating. The horse may then start to look at their sides and paw the ground. You may hear gut sounds initially, since the bowels are working harder to move the impaction through. However, as the condition goes on unresolved, gas will start to build up and pain increases. The gut sounds will then begin to taper off. It is best to keep these horses walking in the early stages as it has been found to enhance gut motility. A short ride in the trailer has shown to be helpful as well. It is thought that the vibration of the trailer gently jostles the abdomen and can relieve gas and promote motility in this manner. Never load a horse that is in a great deal of pain and trying to go down. If the horse must be transported to the clinic, it is best to have a pain medication given to keep the horse stable in transit.

Impaction can be prevented if you know what tends to cause them. One thing to remember is to be sure that the horse's water supply is clean and fresh. Frozen or contaminated water will not be consumed readily thus setting up a drier bowel and increased propensity for impaction. Horses will drink on average 10 gallons of water per 24 hours. On hot days or during exercise this may increase up to 20 gallons. Having fresh water is essential for normal bowel function, keeping the flow of ingesta constant.

Feeding large grain meals once or twice a day has also been shown to increase the risk of impaction. This occurs because the water content inside the bowel will increase and decrease in large swings, setting up for a dehydrated bowel in the down swing. Horses are best adapted to eat small meals all through the day, so if possible try to feed smaller grain meals 3-4 times a day.

Avoid poor quality hays that are high in non-digestible fibers. Coastal Bermuda hay is an example that has been shown to put horses more at risk for an impaction.

Lastly, changing a horse's turn out schedule can alter the gut motility. If a horse is to be stalled for an injury, reduce or eliminate the grain diet and provide good quality high fiber digestible hay. The stalled horse should be walked and allowed to graze a couple times of day if the injury permits.

The treatment of impaction colic is approached medically first. Since the leading factor that may predispose a horse to impaction is a dehydrated bowel, intravenous fluid therapy is usually initiated along with pain medication. Some horses may need as much as 40 liters of fluids to correct the dehydration. The fluids act to re-hydrate the horse as well as promote increased bowel motility. The horse may also benefit from fluid therapy delivered via nasogastric tube every few hours to help hydrate the bowel contents.

If the medical therapy is not effective, surgery may be indicated to remove the impaction. The sooner a horse is treated the better the chance for him to resolve with medical therapy.

## Sand Colic

Horses will naturally have a small amount of sand in their gut. In some areas where the environment may have loose sand in the grazing and feeding areas, horses can ingest too much sand while eating their rations. Over time, if the sand is not eliminated, it can build up and cause problems. Such problems include delayed transit of feed material through the bowel, irritation of the gut lining, and blockage or displacement of the bowel.

Initially, horses with sand colic may only exhibit subtle signs of pain. These include inappetance, finicky eating, stretching out as if to urinate, and spending more time lying down, especially while eating. In some cases, the horse's stool can become loose or resemble a cow patty. Examination of the stool by diluting in a bucket of water can help to reveal the sand in some cases. This is done by collecting the stool off grass or shavings and placing it into a bucket, adding water to break the stool up, waiting an hour or so, and then pouring off the water and floating particles. At the bottom of the bucket you can assess if there is any sand or dirt. More than a tablespoon could be cause for concern. But realize in some cases horses with sand in the gut will not pass sand in every manure pile. Therefore you may have to repeat this test several times if there is sufficient risk for the horse to develop sand colic.

There has been some debate over the best treatment for sand colic. Traditionally, horses may be treated with a psyllium product that can be found at most drug stores. This can be mixed with water and given via nasogastric tube by your vet. The product can also be fed to the horse mixed with water and a concentrate feed. There are also special feed additives made for topdressing the feed to treat sand colic. All in all, the goal is to add highly digestible fiber to the gut to help with motility and water retention. Coarse hay, such as oat hay, is a natural alternative to try as well.

If medical therapy is not successful, surgery may be indicated if the horse's symptoms indicate the colic is worsening. However, as with any surgical endeavor, there can be risk. The quantity of sand in the gut may be large causing the gut wall to be weaker and prone to tearing during manipulation and removal of the sand. This could lead to a potentially fatal infection in the abdomen if the contents of the gut were to spill into the abdominal cavity.

Prevention of sand colic is, of course, the best route to take. If your horse's environment is sandy or the pasture is over-grazed, take these precautions to reduce the risk of sand colic. First, when feeding, keep the food off the ground in a large trough. This eliminates a lot of wasted feed that may otherwise fall on the ground and be nibbled up later. Feed hay on a hard surface such as a rubber mat or on the pasture away from loose dirt and sand. Feed high fiber digestible hays that promote good gut motility and overall health. Supply the horses with a trace mineral block. If your environment is such that you cannot eliminate access to the sandy areas, discuss with your vet the possibility of adding psyllium monthly to your horse's diet.

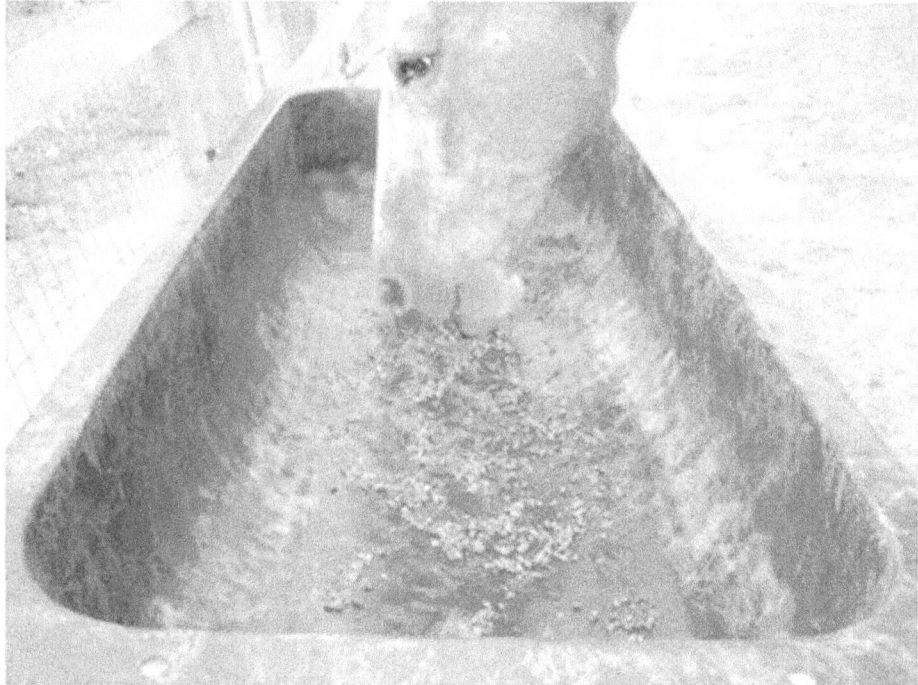

**Figure 6.8:** *Feeding from a trough*

## Strangulating Colic

Colic episodes occur when the bowel is compromised from obstructions either internally, like an impaction, or externally such as a twist or torsion. When the bowel is occluded from an external source such as torsion, hernia, entrapment or displacement, the blood supply to the gut can also be compromised. This can result in a strangulated bowel that will start to die in the segment that has lost blood supply. When the bowel becomes strangulated, and begins to die, poisons from bacteria inside the bowel start to leak out into the abdominal cavity. This results in shock and poor circulation, starting the downward spiral to the death of the horse.

Your physical exam findings will be important to determine signs of shock. Shock can induce a high heart rate (70-90 bpm), high respiration rate, darkened mucous membranes, dehydration and cool extremities, such as the muzzle and ears, due to the poor circulation. Survival from a strangulated bowel requires immediate surgical repair. Even some cases that make it to surgery are euthanized if there is extensive damage involving large sections of intestine.

The diagnosis of a strangulating colic is usually made from a collection of physical and clinical exam findings; amount and frequency of reflux from nasogastric tube, abdominocentesis, rectal examination, and possibly ultrasound examination. These horses are in unrelenting pain and are usually not controllable except with the strongest of pain medications for only short periods of time. If surgery is an option, it should be undertaken as soon as possible.

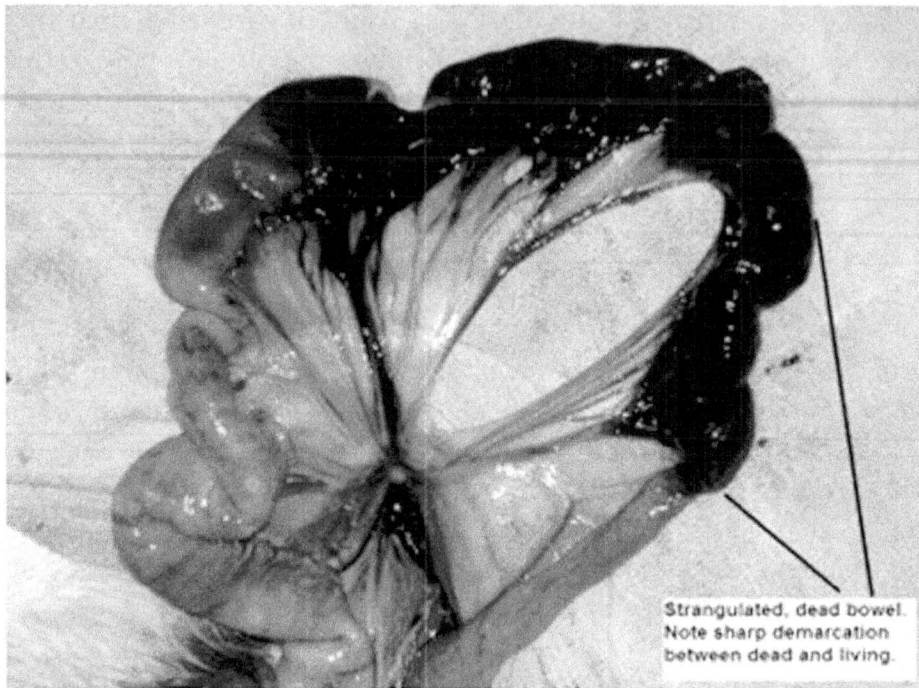

**Figure 6.6:** *Strangulated bowel*

## Grain Overload Colic

In the event that your horse gains access to the feed room or large quantities of grain, there is a risk that the horse will overeat and suffer complications. When you suspect that the horse has overeaten, or you are not sure, the earlier that treatment is instituted the better. Initially, the horse may not show any signs of distress or pain. There may be bloating in the belly and general depression.

Overeating grain can lead to excessive fermentation of the feed in the stomach and the hindgut. The rapid expansion of gases can lead to a stomach rupture if the horse is not decompressed promptly via a nasogastric tube. If the excess grain reaches the lower intestines, toxins from the bacterial fermentation can leach into the bloodstream setting the horse up for endotoxic shock and laminitis or founder from the poisons released into the bloodstream. Treatment is aimed at preventing gas expansion and absorption of the toxins into the bloodstream.

Mineral oil, activated charcoal, and bismuth are used to soak up the toxic fermentation and thereby prevent or at least reduce absorption of these poisons into the bloodstream. These should only be administered via nasogastric tube! Most horses can be started on intravenous fluids and anti-inflammatory medication to get a head start in case they are at risk of laminitis. The sooner you treat the horse, the better the outcome is likely to be. If more than one horse is suspected of eating the grain, they should all be treated respectively.

## Choke (Esophageal obstruction)

Choke in horses is not the same condition as in humans. In people, choke occurs when food or other foreign bodies get lodged in the trachea or windpipe. This is immediately life threatening as asphyxiation can occur unless the obstruction is removed. In horses, choke describes a condition where feed or other material becomes lodged in the esophagus. The horse's air supply is not compromised, but the horse is at risk of aspirating fluid into the lungs while the esophagus is blocked.

Horses that are choked will salivate excessively, cough, and may lie down. Copious amounts of saliva and feed will discharge from the nostrils. Some horses that attempt to swallow while they are choked will exhibit a gag reflex. Many horses will recover spontaneously from choke while others will need to be treated.

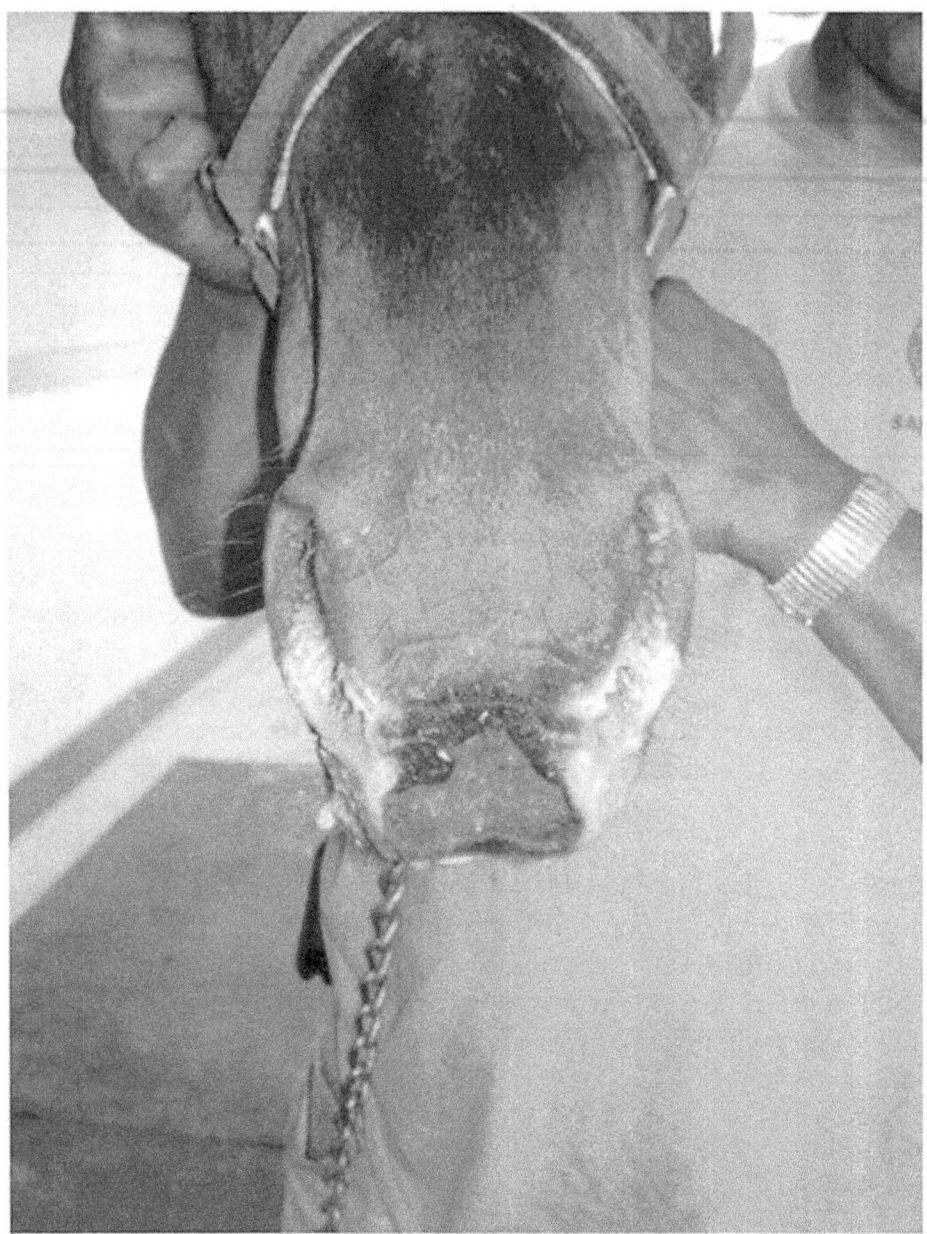

**Figure 6.7:** *Feed at nostrils*

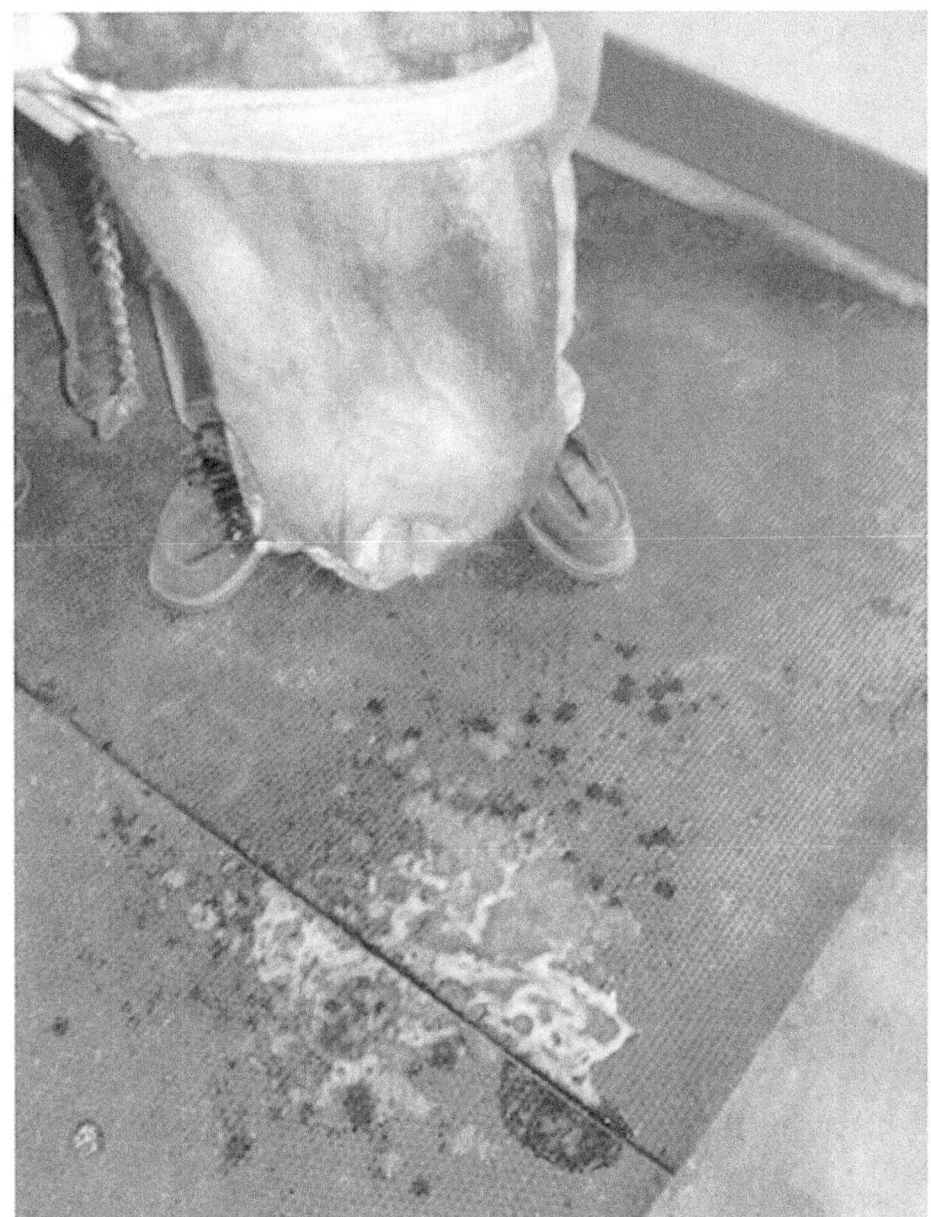

**Figure 6.8:** *Copious discharge from nostrils*

We suggest removing all feed and water. Try walking the horse for 30 minutes, stopping intermittently to massage the left side of the neck.

Massage by starting with your fingers at the lower jaw and keeping pressure while sliding down the neck to the chest. There is a natural groove where your fingers can slide. By massaging in this manner, you may help the obstruction to push through to the stomach. If you watch closely, and notice the horse swallow without a gag reflex, the choke should be cleared. Do not feed the horse anymore feed for the next 12 hours but allow the horse access to water.

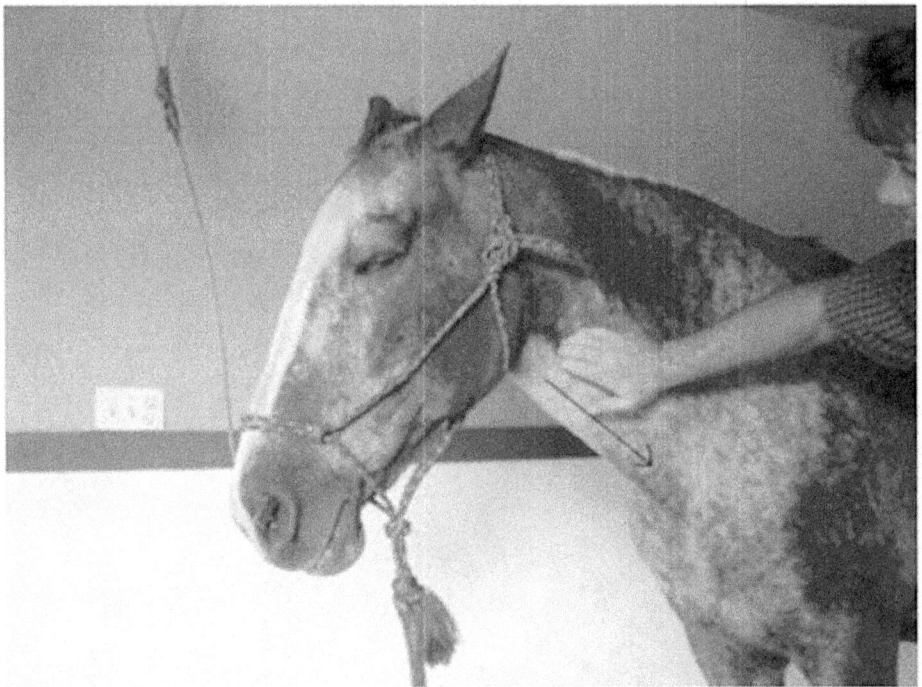

**Figure 6.9a:** *Start choke massage with fingers at lower jaw*

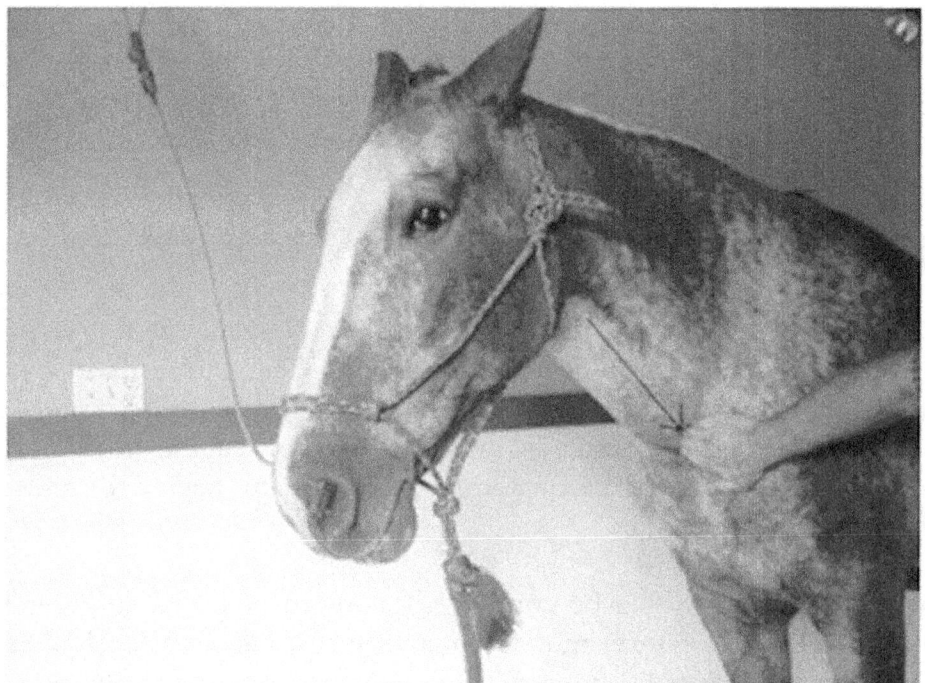

**Figure 6.9b:** *Keep pressure while sliding hand down neck toward chest*

If the choke episode does not pass within 30 min, a veterinarian should be contacted. The horse will be sedated to lower the head while a nasogastric tube is passed to the obstruction. The tube is then flushed and allowed to drain out. Several flushes are usually required to pass the obstruction. In rare cases, the obstruction is a solid object and flushing cannot remove it. In these cases, the horse will be referred to a surgical faculty for an endoscopic and/or radiographic exam. Be sure to examine the horse's teeth while they are sedated. Sometimes poor dentition is a culprit for choke.

You may also prevent choke by spreading the horse's feed over a larger surface area such as a trough. This prevents the horse from bolting the feed, and swallowing without chewing thoroughly. Placing a large stone or salt brick in the feed bucket may also slow the horse down while they eat.

After a horse recovers from choke, the following feedings should be moistened. Careful auscultation of the lungs with a stethoscope should be performed to rule out any chance of secondary aspiration pneumonia. In some cases, when aspiration is a risk, the horse will be started on antibiotic therapy.

## Diarrhea

Diarrhea is caused when the fluid in the large intestine is not resorbed back into the body before leaving the rectum. This can result in a softer stool or a stool without any consistency at all, resembling water. All cases of diarrhea can result in rapid dehydration of the horse. In all cases the horse should be quarantined since many bacterial agents are the source of disease.

A physical exam should be completed taking into special consideration the horse's temperature, mucous membranes, skin tent for hydration, and heart rate. Gut sounds will most likely be elevated as the bowel is irritated and hypermotile.

Confine the horse to a stall if possible and do not allow anyone but the primary caretaker(s) to handle the horse in order to prevent spread of bacterial agents. Place a foot bath outside the stall with 50% bleach and water to disinfect your feet. Wash hands after treating affected animals.

Affected horses should be evaluated by your vet to determine the causal agent of the diarrhea if possible, and to initiate antibiotic and fluid therapy if needed. Keep the water supply fresh to encourage drinking. Adding electrolytes to a second bucket of water is also helpful to offer as a free choice supplement. Bacterial cultures of the stool can be helpful in determining the cause of the diarrhea. These cultures should be obtained before antibiotics are administered.

## Ulcers

Ulceration of the stomach is not an uncommon condition in young horses, especially those that may be under stress from training or illness. It is worthwhile to mention in this chapter since it deals with the GI tract. However, stomach ulceration is not a sudden emergency situation. It is usually a gradual onset with a decrease in appetite, pawing the ground on occasion, grinding teeth and showing minor colic symptoms sometimes while eating a grain meal.

Stomach ulceration is not necessarily a life threatening condition, but prompt diagnosis is important to limit the amount of damage to the stomach. Several therapies are available to treat as well as prevent stomach ulceration. It will depend on the severity of the problem as to which medications should be used to treat the horse.

To accurately assess the extent of ulceration, an endoscopic exam can be performed to visualize the stomach lining. Omeprazole is one of the leading treatments available and one of the most effective at this time. Ulcer treatment with omeprazole can be costly--a 4 week supply could range $800-$1200.

## Conclusion

Having a good knowledge of your horse's gastrointestinal system is paramount for the horse owner. Sudden shifts in diet can be extremely detrimental. Nutritional additives that may advertise weight gain or better hair coats, etc. are no replacement for good quality hay, pasture, and grain products. If a change is to be made in the horse's diet or even turn out, make it gradual so as not to induce a colic episode. Treat colic early and notify your vet at the onset of symptoms to start a timeline for treatment and progress. Keep your trailer in good repair in the event you have to transport in an emergency.

# Respiratory Emergencies

CHAPTER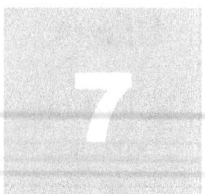

Respiratory conditions that can lead to disease will usually be noticed by a discharge from one or both nostrils, respiratory distress, and/or audible wheezing. A respiratory emergency is not common in that you would come home and suddenly find your horse with pneumonia and call the vet after hours. Instead, diseases of the lower respiratory tract or the lungs normally will have a gradual onset. Diseases of the upper respiratory tract can come on gradually or may have a sudden onset as with allergic reactions, acute infections, or venomous bites to the muzzle. This chapter will cover those emergencies of the upper respiratory tract first followed by emergencies of the lower tract.

## Upper Respiratory

The upper respiratory tract is composed of the nostrils, nasal sinuses, guttural pouches, larynx, and trachea. Many diseases can affect these structures, ranging from infections, allergies, trauma, and in some cases cancer. Horses with acute upper respiratory disease will often make noise while breathing. Typically this may be a wheeze or rattling noise during the inspiration or breathing in phase. Many of these horses will be quite distressed as there is an urgency to breathe. Try to keep them calm, avoid any exertion that would increase oxygen demand. Notify your vet at once and describe the symptoms. If the horse's breathing is becoming more and more labored in a short period of time, an emergency tracheotomy may need to be performed.

### Airway Obstruction

The clinical signs of a horse in respiratory distress are not hard to notice. These horses are literally fighting for air to breathe. They will be extremely distressed and often collapse without warning if the airway is not opened. Although the causes for airway obstruction are numerous, you need not try to decipher why the airway has become obstructed. Instead, take quick measures to establish an airway and stabilize the horse.

If the airway is obstructed at the nostrils due to swelling, you will need to insert a tube into one of the nostrils to allow airflow. Horses are not readily capable of breathing through their mouths. Therefore, any obstruction to the nostrils can cause suffocation. For example, a venomous snake bite to the muzzle can cause enough swelling to impede breathing. In a vicious cycle, the horse will struggle more and more to breathe, causing turbulent air flow to only increase the swelling. Waiting for your vet to arrive could prove fatal to the horse.

Cut a section of small 1/2 to 3/4 inch diameter hose at a length of 8-12 inches depending on the size of the horse. Lubricate the hose with whatever is close by--hand lotion, Vaseline or just water. Insert into either nostril to a depth of approximately 8 inches. If possible, try to direct the tube downward while inserting. Obviously the distressed horse is going to put up some rejection to this procedure. But if the horse is truly lacking oxygen, and on the verge of collapse, there will be little struggle. Be aware that bleeding from the nose may occur. If the horse is breathing easier, the bleeding will stop in a few minutes.

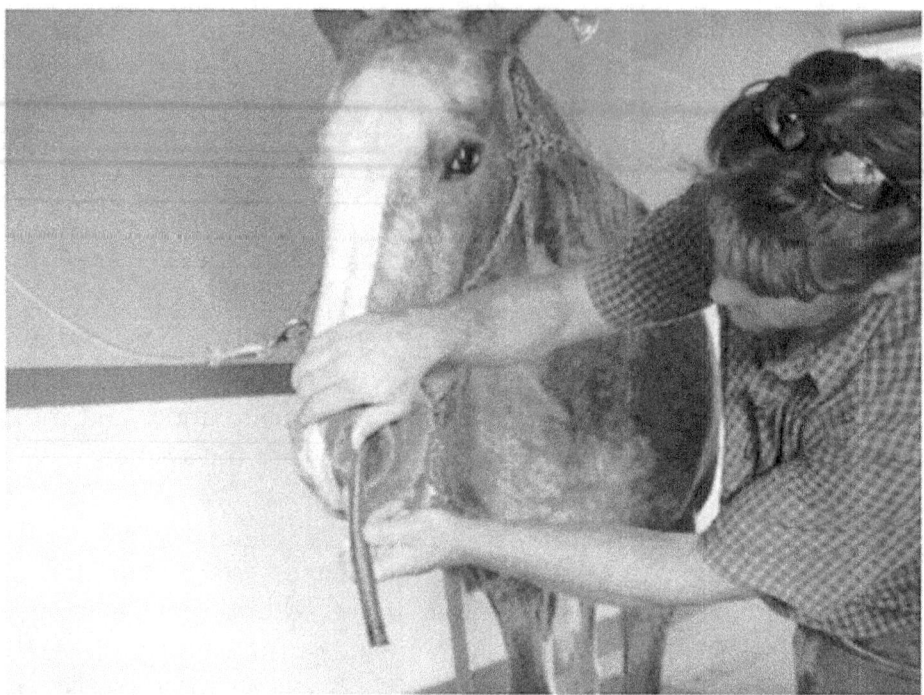

**Figure 7.1:** *Insertion of 8 inch tube for obstructed airway*

The airway may also become obstructed near the larynx or in the trachea. Situations such as anaphylaxis that causes edema or swelling in the trachea could lead to near complete obstruction of the trachea. When alerting your veterinarian to this type of respiratory emergency, advise them that a tracheotomy tube may be needed. Better safe than sorry! A tracheotomy is performed to establish an airway in patients that cannot be intubated, which means to have a tube passed from the nostril or mouth into trachea. Tracheotomies are left in place until the offending swelling is under control. Below is a list of conditions that could require the need for tracheotomy:

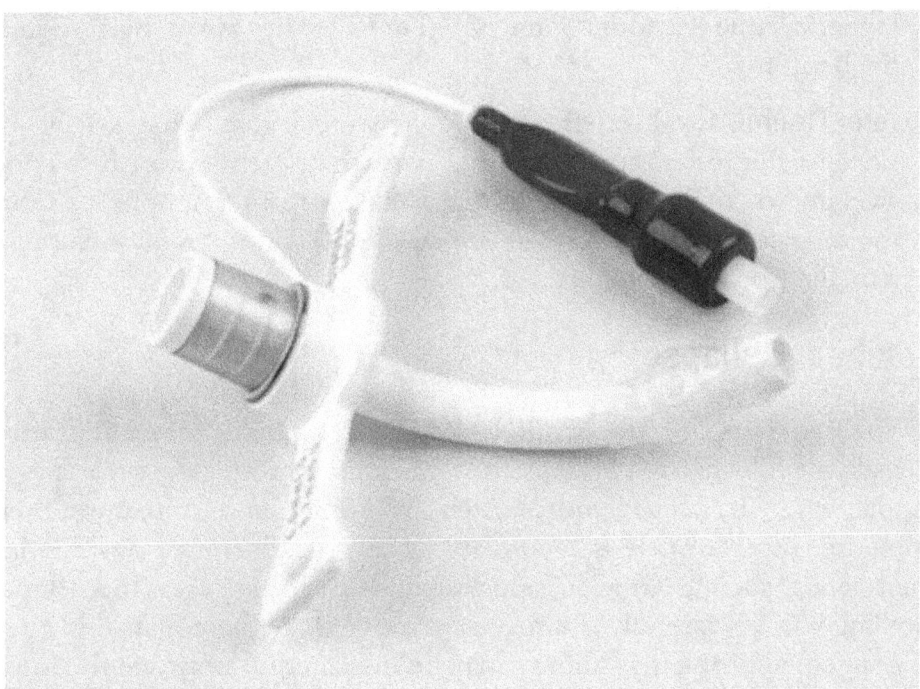

**Figure 7.2:** *Tracheotomy tube*

**Anaphylaxis.** Anaphylaxis describes a severe immune reaction to a foreign substance such as insect stings, vaccines, some food products, and numerous drugs. Treatment with epinephrine is needed immediately to reverse the immune reaction. Multiple body systems affected, but the swelling in the trachea can lead to life-threatening suffocation.

**Strangles with Severe Lymph Node Swelling.** This can occur in foals and yearlings afflicted with strangles. Strangles is the laymen term for a highly contagious upper airway bacterial disease. The lymph nodes around the pharynx can become engorged with pus, thereby impeding airflow in the trachea. A tracheotomy is needed in these cases until the lymph nodes can be drained or reduced in size.

**Laryngeal Paralysis.** If only one side of the larynx is paralyzed you will hear a roaring sound at exercise. In the rare case of full paralysis of the trachea from toxins or other metabolic conditions such as

Hyperkalemic Periodic Paralysis (HYPP), the horse may require a tracheotomy.

**Severe Trauma to Muzzle/Face.** Any severe trauma that affects both sides of the muzzle or face could have the potential to cause enough swelling to compromise breathing. Snake or other venomous bites to the muzzle may also cause severe swelling. If this situation is present, a tracheotomy may be needed.

## Tracheal Collapse

As the name implies, the windpipe of affected horses may intermittently partially or fully close. Affected horses exhibit a respiratory noise as well as distress. It occurs more often in ponies and miniature breeds. Sometimes the collapse is secondary to an outside source pushing in on the trachea, such as an abscess or a mass. In these cases, the offending swelling can be carefully drained or removed. If the collapse is a result of congenital problems, surgery may be indicated to improve the internal diameter of the trachea. Fortunately, tracheal collapse is uncommon.

## Esophageal Choke

Choke of this nature defines an obstruction within the esophagus. Due to the inability to swallow normally, excessive saliva is refluxed back up into the mouth and nasal cavity. Affected horses will cough and have feed material mixed with saliva flowing from both nostrils. In such cases there is a risk of the horse aspirating or breathing in the saliva and feed material into the trachea and lungs.

Horses that have esophageal choke should be sedated to lower the head, thereby decreasing the chance of feed material and saliva flowing down the trachea. Once sedated, a tube is passed and the obstruction is flushed out of the esophagus. A thorough exam of the chest with a stethoscope is performed to ensure no fluid has been aspirated. If needed the horse may be started on antibiotic therapy. Refer to Chapter 6 for a full description of esophageal choke.

## Shipping Fever (upper and lower respiratory)

Shipping fever is a generic term used to describe several common respiratory conditions in horses and other livestock. These diseases may be viral or bacterial in nature or both. Horses do not necessarily have to be shipped to come down with disease. Although the process of shipping and transport in a truck or trailer predisposes the horse to stress factors which can lead to disease.

These stress factors include crowding with other horses, poor ventilation, increased dust levels and fatigue. Before you ship your horse, be sure to perform a thorough exam including a temperature reading to make sure they are healthy for the trip. A slight viral infection that would otherwise run a course after a couple days could progress to pneumonia if the horse were to be shipped.

If your horse has arrived at their destination with a fever and nasal discharge, try to reduce stress by keeping them in a warm, dry environment isolated from other horses. Institute the appropriate antibiotic therapy as prescribed by your veterinarian. Flunixin or Phenylbutazone may be needed to reduce a fever so the horse will resume eating.

## Strangles

Strangles is a highly contagious disease of equines that has worldwide distribution. The causative organism is a Streptococcus bacterium similar to the bacterium that causes strep throat in people. Clinically, horses will exhibit high fever 105F or greater, depression, thick nasal discharge, and lymph node swelling around the throat and mandibles.

Younger horses never exposed to strangles typically develop the upper respiratory form. Older horses may develop purpura hemorrhagica from exposure to strangles. This is characterized by fever, swelling in the legs and lower abdomen, and possibly hives. Purpura can be a life threatening disease especially if the swelling is associated with the trachea.

If strangles is suspected, immediately isolate the affected horse(s). The clothing and shoes of any handler and the equipment associated with those horses can carry the infectious bacteria. One person should be assigned to their care to avoid spread throughout the farm.

Although the use of antibiotics is controversial in the treatment of strangles, discuss this with your veterinarian. There may also be a need for anti-inflammatory medication to reduce swelling and fever. If the lymph nodes are severely swollen around the larynx, an emergency tracheotomy may be needed to establish an airway. Avoid stressing these compromised horses until your vet arrives.

## Snake Bite/Blunt trauma to muzzle

Since horses usually have their head down most of the time while out to pasture, the muzzle is a common place to be bitten. Depending on the type of snake and the amount of venom delivered, swelling can be moderate to severe. Initially, the muzzle will swell and be warm. Later, the muzzle may become cool as the tissue begins to die from the venom toxins.

If there is immediate obstruction to airflow, insert a short tube or other object such as an open syringe case to prevent complete closure of the nostrils. Your veterinarian may wish to prescribe anti-inflammatory medication to further decrease the swelling. Try to keep the horse's head elevated to keep the swelling to a minimum as well. Since the venom is very toxic to tissue, a local area of necrosis or tissue death will likely occur. For this reason antibiotic therapy is indicated. Do not use ice or attempt to suction the venom out. These procedures are not effective.

Blunt trauma to the muzzle could also cause substantial swelling. The initial treatment to reduce swelling and provide an airway after blunt trauma is similar to the treatment described above for snakebite to the muzzle.

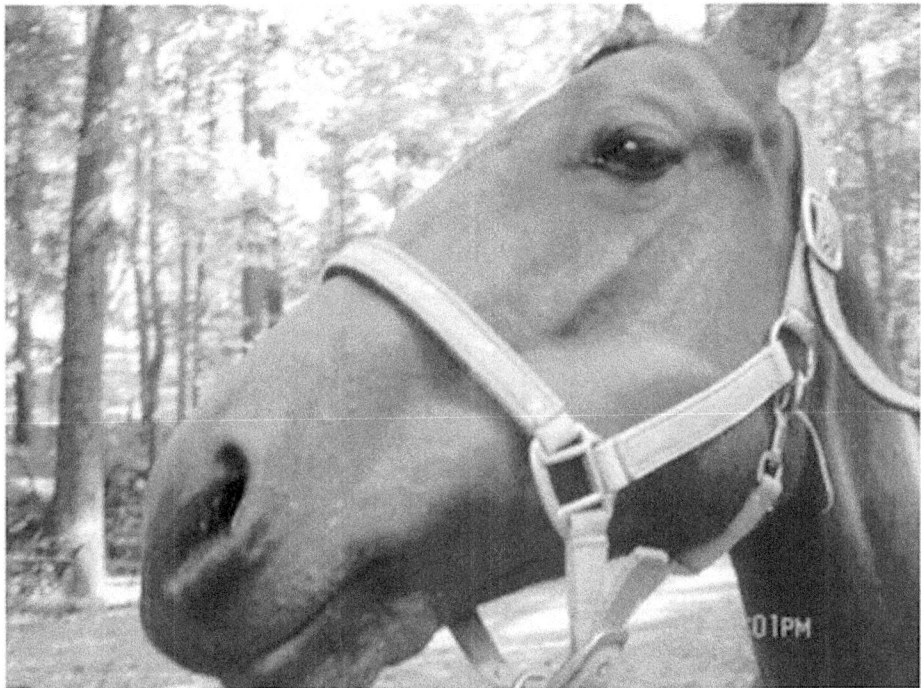

**Figure 7.1** *Venomous snake bite to mandible and cheek area*

## Epistaxis

Epistaxis is a medical term that describes a nosebleed. Nosebleeds can occur from the placement of a tube into the delicate nasal cavity. These are self-limiting and will normally clot within 10 -15 minutes or less. The following is a list of several other causes for bleeds:

**Ethmoid hematoma**. A mass that grows deep within the nasal cavity. Blood is usually from one side of the nostril and mixed with other secretions. Diagnosis is based on endoscopes and/or radiographs of the head. Ethmoid hematomas may be treated by injections of formalin and/or laser treatment.

- **Guttural pouch mycosis.** The guttural pouch is a unique cavity located deep in the horse's pharynx area. Within the cavity are several cranial nerves and large arteries. Fungal infections can cause severe erosions in the area leading to bleeding and neurological dysfunction.

- **Bleeding disorder.** As in humans, horses can have bleeding disorders where the platelets, which are responsible for blood clotting, are severely depleted. Blood work is necessary in order to determine if this is the cause.

- **Exercised-Induced Pulmonary Hemmorhage.** This is typically a disease of race horses. Bleeding occurs within the lungs. Rarely is blood seen at the nostrils.

- **Tooth Abscess - Upper cheek teeth only.** One-sided drainage will consist of blood tinged pink with putrid odor. A thorough oral exam, possibly with radiographs, is needed to determine the extent of the infection. Surgical removal of the tooth and treatment of the affected sinus cavity is necessary to resolve the problem.

Nose bleeds should be addressed and evaluated, but rarely on an emergency basis. If bleeding is profuse, and will not slow down after 10-15 minutes, the problem should be addressed by your veterinarian. Running a cool stream of water over the bridge of the nose and/or placing an ice pack behind the ears can be helpful in some cases. Keep the horse quiet and still. Remember an 1,100 lb horse has roughly 11 gallons of blood circulating in their body. They can lose 1.5 to 2 gallons before life threatening shock may occur.

# Lower Respiratory

Lower respiratory disease describes problems with lungs, the lining of the chest cavity and the diaphragm. During your initial exam pay attention to the inspiration and expiration phases of breathing. When a horse is suffering from lower respiratory disease as opposed to upper respiratory disease, the expiratory phase is usually labored. While listening with your stethoscope you may hear wheezing and crackling in the chest. A trained ear is needed in some cases to distinguish normal sounds from abnormal. Contact you vet if you feel unsure of your findings. Some horses with pneumonia may have little to no outward signs of disease. Therefore, a thorough exam of the chest with a stethoscope is needed to determine whether a problem exists.

## Recurrent Airway Obstruction (RAO)/Heaves

This is a disease that was previously referred to as Chronic Obstructive Pulmonary Disease (COPD). There are basically two forms of the disease. One occurs in stabled horses that react to organic dusts and molds from hay and other particulates found in higher concentrations inside buildings such as barns. Another form is termed Summer Pasture Associated Obstructive Pulmonary Disease (SPAOD). Horses suffering from this form typically live in the southeastern states. Signs are worse when these animals are on pastures during hot humid weather.

Horses afflicted with either form of disease show varying signs depending on the severity and the stage of disease and if the horse is experiencing a recurring episode. Initially, there may be a cough or just milky nasal discharge. This is usually incited during high dust times such as feeding and cleaning the barn. Some horses may cough when starting to exercise. Progressive symptoms include nasal flaring and obvious respiratory difficulty. You may notice the horse using abdominal muscles to force out their air when breathing. In advanced cases, you may see all the latter signs in addition to loss of appetite and audible wheezing.

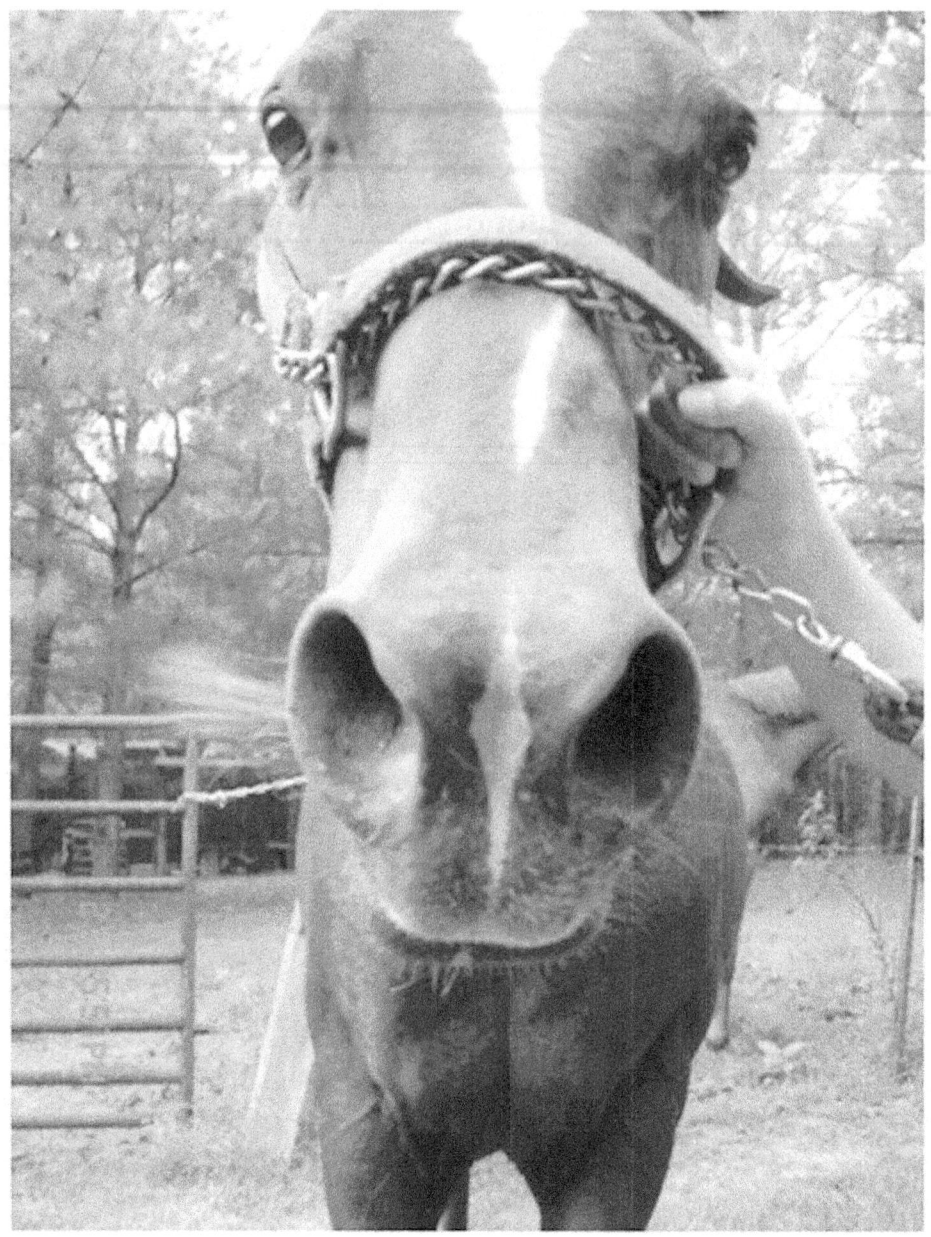

**Figure 7.2:** *Nostril flare*

Management of the horse's environment is a big part of the treatment for RAO/SPAOD. Maintaining a strict, low dust, environment for

RAO affected horses is paramount. This means for RAO horses, staying outdoors all the time. Even brief exposure of just minutes inside the barn could initiate an episode. Select feeds and beddings that have low dust content for both RAO and SPAOD horses. Wetting the hay down can be beneficial as well.

In the event your horse has been diagnosed with RAO or SPAOD, your veterinarian may decide to treat the horse medically in addition to environmental modifications. For acute outbreaks, your veterinarian may leave you with a corticosteroid and/or bronchodilator drug. These drugs may be administered via injection, oral, or inhalation methods. If your horse suffers an acute severe attack, atropine can be administered via IV by your veterinarian to quell the bronchospasms. Overuse of atropine can have detrimental effects on intestinal function such as slowing down or stopping GI tract motion.

What is best for your horse will be determined by the severity of the condition and how well the environment can be modified to suit the horse's needs. It should also be noted that allergy testing along with desensitization therapy has shown to be of benefit for some horses.

## Pleuropneumonia - Pleuritis and Pleurisy

This disease describes an inflammation and/or infection of the pleural membranes. The pleural membrane is the interior lining of the chest. It also covers the lungs as a very thin membrane. In horses, pleuritis can occur without involvement of the lung, but in most cases the pleuritis is secondary to a primary lung infection or pneumonia.

Affected horses may be reluctant to move, hold their elbows away from their chest, stop eating, develop fever and exhibit shallow and labored breathing. With the stethoscope, abnormal lung sounds are usually present on the lower right side. Several methods may be employed to definitely diagnose a horse with pleuropneumonia.

A non-invasive approach to diagnosis utilizes auscultation with the stethoscope as well as ultrasound of the chest. Fluid present in the pleural cavity can be obtained and cultured for bacteria. An aggressive regimen of treatment with chest drainage, if necessary, as well as appropriate antibiotic therapy should be started at once if pleuritis has been diagnosed. These horses will be best managed in a hospital environment unless the initial transport there would prove too stressful. Long term therapy is often needed for survival.

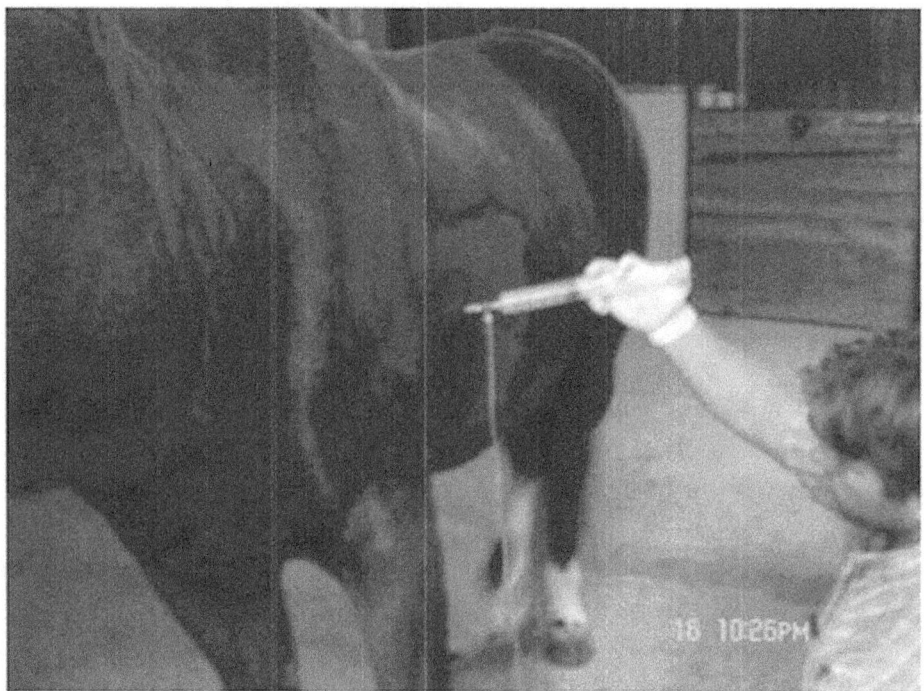

**Figure 7.3:** *Thoracocentesis*

## Aspiration Pneumonia

Aspiration pneumonia occurs when foreign solid or liquid material is inhaled into the lungs. Depending upon the amount and infectious quality of the material, aspiration pneumonia can cause life threatening or short-term disease. In horses, aspiration pneumonia can be common after esophageal choke. With the stethoscope you may hear a loud gurgling or fluttering sound in the lower front part of the chest. This is the same area where you would normally listen for the heart. Be sure to listen from both sides. After several hours, the respiratory sounds may turn to crackles and wheezes. Prompt treatment with antibiotics and anti-inflammatory medication is advised. Fortunately, most horses that experience aspiration pneumonia secondary to esophageal choke do well.

## Rhodococcus equi Pneumonia (Foal)

This is a disease of young foals typically between the ages of 2 weeks to 4 months. The disease usually occurs quickly and can affect several animals on the farm. Since the organism responsible for disease comes from the environment, it is likely that other foals may have been affected on the same farm in the past. For this reason, some farms elect to treat foals with a preventative antiserum if there is a history of Rhodococcus infections from the past.

The causative bacteria survive well in the environment and resist harsh, dry climates. Affected foals are generally febrile or with fever, off-feed, unthrifty in appearance, and may exhibit a moist cough. Examination with a stethoscope can reveal harsh crackles in the lung fields. Multiple small abscesses develop within the lungs that may be detected with radiographs. Definitive diagnosis may be obtained from culture of the fluid from a tracheal wash.

## Pneumothorax/Chest Trauma

Pneumothorax is a condition that occurs when the pleural cavity begins to fill with air. The pleural cavity normally contains only a slight amount of fluid. Pneumothorax can occur when there is trauma to the chest from the exterior that allows air to be sucked in from the outside. Any deep wound to the chest area could potentially cause pneumothorax. The wound may exhibit a sucking sound. If so, there is a high probability that the horse could develop pneumothorax. The resulting air in the pleural space could cause the lung on the affected side to collapse. Horses will show obvious signs of respiratory difficulty and lung sounds on the affected side will be absent when listening with a stethoscope.

There are diagnostic procedures that your veterinarian can perform to determine if pneumothorax is truly present. Pneumothorax can also arise secondary to pneumonia. At any rate, there is a serious risk of death if the problem is not resolved quickly. The patient should be stabilized, wounds should be sutured and the air in the chest should be removed as soon as possible.

Affected horse should be placed on broad spectrum antibiotics. If your horse has suffered a deep chest wound, and you hear air sucking, cover the wound to prevent any more air from being sucked into the chest wall

## Synchronous Diaphragmatic Flutter (Thumps)

Synchronous diaphragmatic flutter (SDF) describes a condition where the nerve that supplies the diaphragm, which is the sheet of muscle responsible for normal breathing, is over-sensitive to stimulation. The nerve, called the phrenic nerve, becomes linked with the electrical activity of the heart and causes a synchronous contraction of the diaphragm with every heartbeat. It may appear to resemble hiccups or hiccoughs. The sensitivity of the phrenic nerve is over-enhanced due to electrolyte imbalances. These imbalances occur in horses that endure strenuous exercise usually over a long period of time. Dehydration tends to occur and the normal electrolyte balance is skewed. In particular, the calcium content is dropped. Therapy involves replacement of necessary electrolytes including calcium and re-hydration. SDF is not considered a fatal disease. Mares that are in heavy lactation can experience SDF due to low circulating levels of calcium. SDF is a rare condition.

## Smoke Inhalation

It is hard to imagine the panic a horse must endure when trapped inside a burning barn. The only hope is that a human will intervene and extricate the horse or they will break out themselves. In the event a horse is rescued from a burning barn with or without burns to the skin, there is a risk the horse will suffer from smoke inhalation. As with people, there are serious side effects that go along with smoke inhalation in horses.

If you have rescued your horse(s) from a fire, do a quick external exam for burns. Burns will be discussed in another chapter. If there are no apparent burns, next address the horse's respiration. Is it labored or shallow? Is there a cough or any discharge from the nostrils? Is the gum color not pink? If you answer yes to any of these questions, contact a veterinarian in order to initiate medical therapy.

These horses are at risk of developing pulmonary edema, a life threatening condition when fluid begins to build up within the lung tissues. Similarly, these horses are also prone to developing pneumonia. For this reason they may actually benefit from hospitalization where shock therapy can be initiated. Affected horses may require oxygen and fluid therapy, anti-inflammatory medication, bronchodilators, and broad spectrum antibiotics.

# Conclusion

Respiratory emergencies constitute a smaller percentage of overall emergency situations. In a pinch, you should be prepared to establish an airway or keep an airway open through the nostril until help arrives. Become familiar with contagious respiratory disease to avoid spread amongst healthy horses. Follow the guidelines of care for the horse with RAO. Avoid environments that could trigger an episode of RAO. Finally, hone your exam skills so that in the event you do need emergency assistance, you may alert your vet that a tracheotomy may need to be performed or oxygen might be needed. These small details can make large differences in the overall outcome of your emergency.

# Trauma Emergencies

CHAPTER

## Lameness and Injuries

Most everything that surrounds a horse's daily routine can lead to trauma. Undoubtedly, one of the most common emergency calls that I will handle deals with trauma. The injury may be a laceration, a broken bone, or acute severe lameness. Certain factors such as the horse's instinctive response to danger, as well as the environmental surroundings of horses contribute to reasons why these animals tend to be predisposed to trauma.

Equine nature is that of a flight-type animal. Just as lions are predators and zebras are the prey, people are sometimes the predators and horses are the prey. Some horses would rather bolt away from a plastic bag even though they may be going through a barb wire fence to get away from the deadly bag! This response is programmed into their genetic make-up. We can assess that the bag is not a hazard, whereas the horse would not take the chance. Instead, a horse will flee away and then, at a safer distance, turn around and snort a time or two while taking that second look at the bag.

Although there appears to be disadvantages for this flight-type response, it actually is advantageous for the horse overall. In fact, it has helped them to evolve over millions of years. The flight-type response is really only problematic from a human perspective. I have yet to hear a horse tell me that they wished they were not so flighty. Horses are put into unusual environments and asked to go into small cramped spaces that they would not naturally be inclined to go. The fact that horses do some of these unnatural tasks is amazing, and reiterates their trust in us humans! It may seem like a safe stall or fenced pasture with all the necessary precautions, but it is not the natural environment to be in during the instinctive response when horses feel trapped and scared. For example, I wonder how many horses get cast in the wild? For all we put them through, it is amazing they come out unscathed in many instances! So we have domesticated these great and noble creatures, now we must tend to those almost inevitable injuries.

## Skin

Horses are not gifted with tough thick hides like cattle. They are therefore more apt to lacerations if caught in a bad situation. We need to be prepared to handle these emergencies. Complete textbooks have been written on the subject of equine skin. The scope in this section of trauma will only be limited to skin emergencies. We start here by giving a brief description of the purpose of skin and what emergencies you may encounter.

The skin is the largest organ. The most important functions are protection from outside infection and thermoregulation. As mentioned earlier, horses have thin skin when compared to other large animals. For this reason, trauma is more likely to occur when struck by objects.

## Lacerations

If you own or care for horses, it is almost inevitable that you will have to contend with a laceration at some point. Mild or severe, you still need to know what to do initially. Cleaning a wound properly is important. A clean wound is imperative is suturing needs to be performed. Also, a clean wound lessens the likelihood that an infection will develop. There are many cleansing agents available, your choice should include one that kills bacteria, is non-irritating, and has some residual effect.

If the wound is in a tough area to clean or the horse is uncomfortable with the procedure, wait until the horse can be sedated. This allows for a much more thorough exam as well as deeper cleaning. Remember the first aid kit from chapter one? Well, now you get to use it. Inside you should find a bottle of normal saline (0.9% NaCl), chlorhexadine scrub

(Nolvasan™) and gauze sponges. Using tap water is fine although it may sting more. Normal saline matches the tissue's fluid content so there is less burn. Change sponges often when washing a wound. Using the same washcloth or rag can re-contaminate the wound and may even drive contamination deeper into the wound. Avoid the use of hydrogen peroxide. I know people like the fizzing and bubbling that occurs when it is poured over a wound. However, it is quite irritating to healthy tissue and should be avoided as a cleanser. It is fine to use for removing excessive or dried blood from the surrounding skin.

Lastly, after the wound is clean, apply salve with an antibiotic ointment with or without a bandage. You now must determine whether the wound needs veterinary attention or can be managed as an open wound. A call to your veterinarian to describe the location of the wound is advised especially if there is a risk of damage to deeper structures.

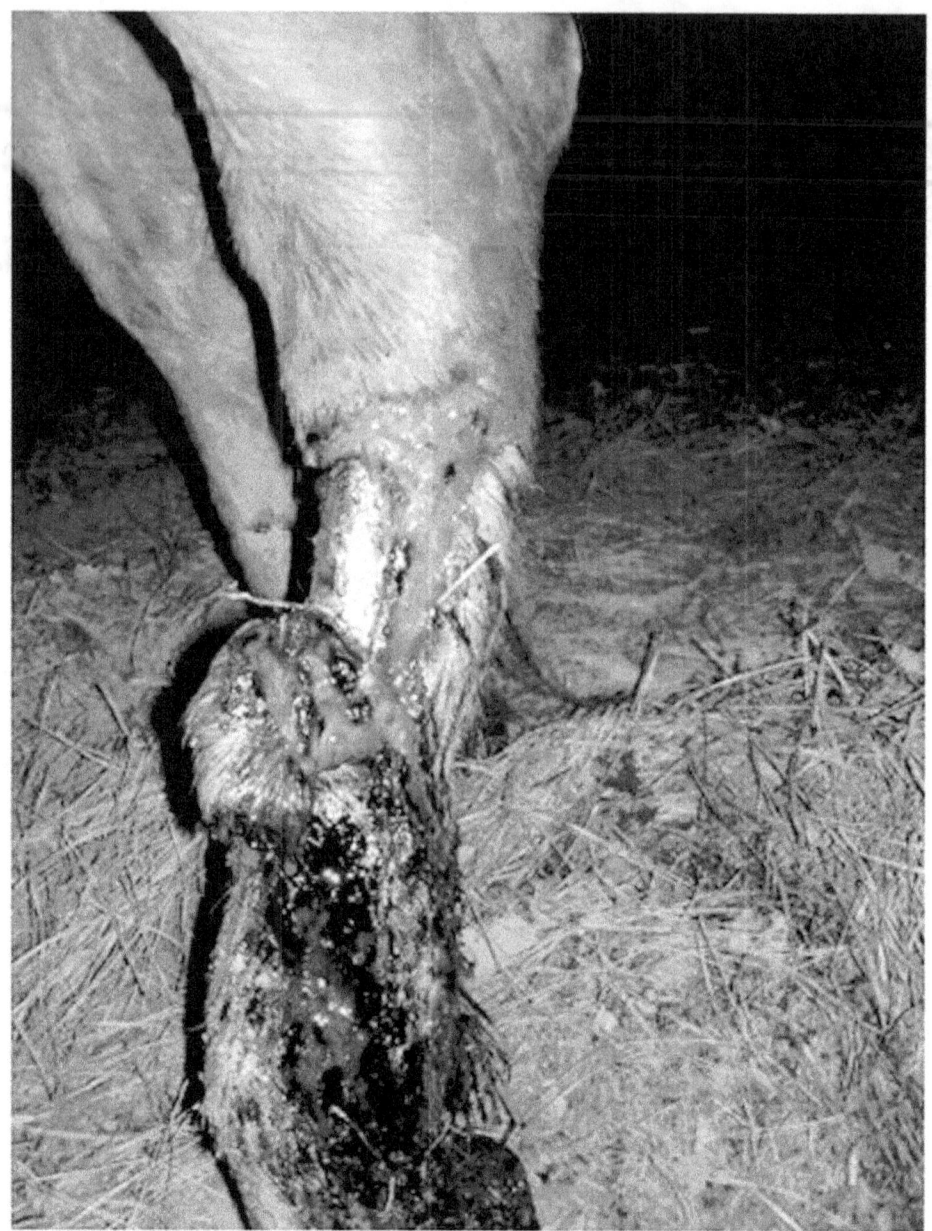

**Figure 8.1:** *Severe laceration to hindlimb*

## Bleeding

Many people panic at the site of blood. More people panic at the quantity of blood loss. As mentioned before, an 1,100 lb horse will have roughly 11 gallons of blood circulating in their body. They can stand to lose 1.5 to 2 gallons before there is a risk of shock or collapse. Large vessels and arteries can be involved in lacerations and will pose a life threatening dilemma if the bleeding is not brought under control quickly.

As with any animal that is experiencing uncontrolled bleeding, application of pressure either by hand or bandage is the primary goal. Cleaning the wound is not the first priority if bleeding is profuse. With leg wounds, application of a cotton or quilted pad together with a polo wrap or VetWrap™ is usually sufficient to slow the bleeding. Quiet the horse and try to limit movement.

If the horse can remain quiet, the bleeding will slow or even clot. Tourniquets should not be applied by inexperienced people. More damage to tendons and other tissues can occur if the tourniquet is applied inappropriately or left in place too long. Assess your horse's vital signs for impending problems from the blood loss. An increased heart rate, a weaker/thready pulse and pale gums indicate large blood loss.

## Tendon Lacerations

Tendons of the lower legs can be divided into two general categories; extensors on the front of all four limbs, and flexors on the rear of all four limbs. It is more common to have injuries occur to the extensor tendons, especially on the hind limb. The back limb typically gets caught between fence board or wire, then the horse jerks the leg quickly causing the laceration to flap down usually just below the hock.

Fortunately, extensor tendon lacerations have a better prognosis for recovery as opposed to flexor tendon lacerations. In many cases, the extensor tendons can repair themselves over time with scar tissue and tendon ends reuniting. In the early stages, a horse with extensor tendon lacerations will tend to knuckle over on the affected foot. They may also drag the foot, not having the ability to flip it forward with each stride. Often a good support wrap or splint is all that is needed to assist in the early stages of healing. Eventually these horses will fill in the defect area with scar tissue that strengthens the limb and allows for a normal stride.

Flexor tendon lacerations can be life threatening. On the rear of the front and hind limbs there is a group of three tendons that are essentially stacked on each other. Starting closest to the skin is the superficial flexor, next is the deep digital flexor, and last is the suspensory ligament. Obvious deformities occur following ruptured or lacerated flexor tendons. A drop in the fetlock joint is typically seen with any of the three tendons involved. Rocking back on the heel with the toe rising up off the ground can be seen with lacerations to the deep flexor tendon.

Repair to these tendons can be performed, but bear in mind that infection of the tendon sheath is a potential problem during healing. Furthermore, subsequent laminitis in the opposite limb can occur if the horse does not resume normal and equal weight-bearing in a short period of time.

If lacerations to either the extensors or flexors are suspected, provide a heavy support wrap to immobilize the limb. Be sure the bandage extends to the foot. Contact your veterinarian.

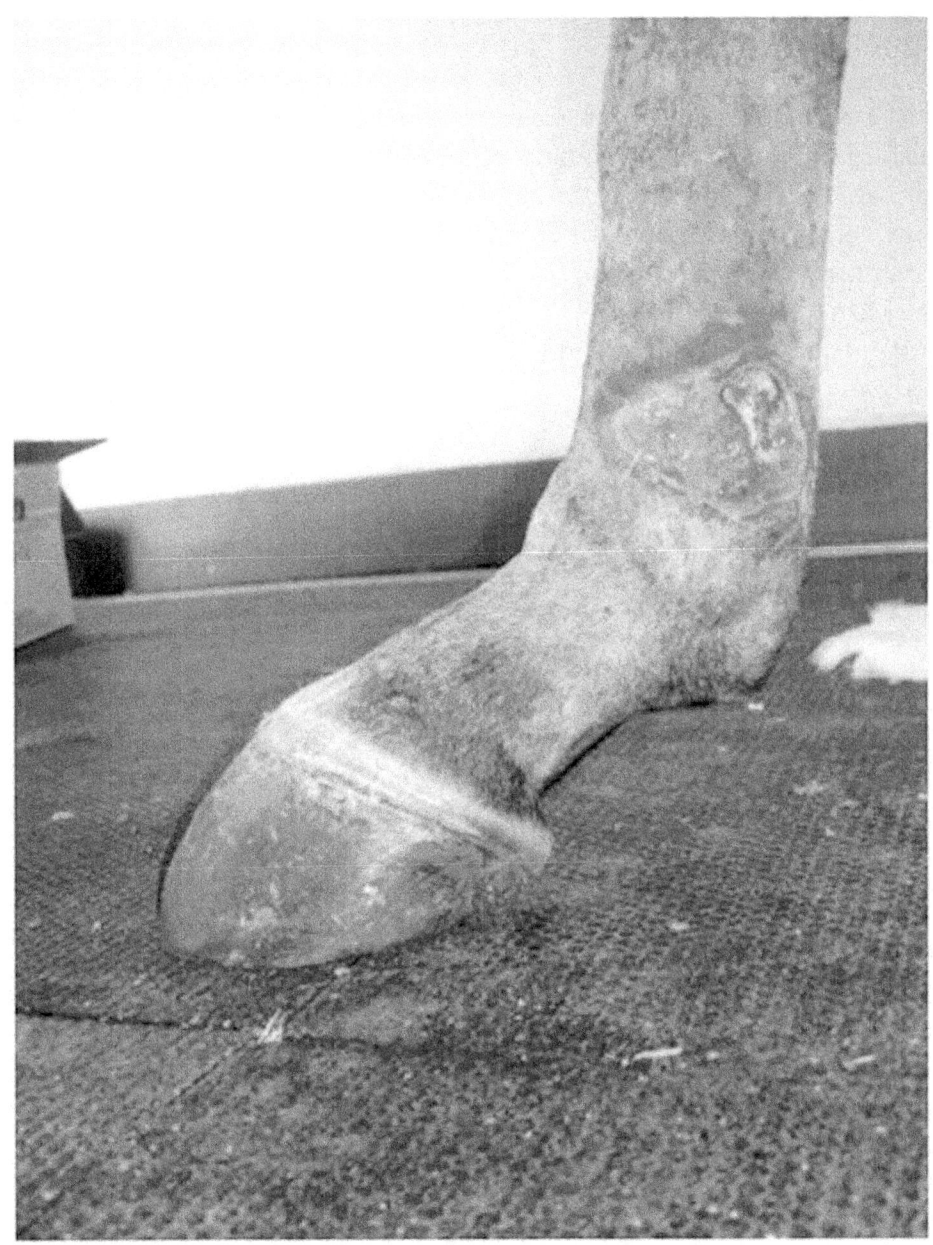

**Figure 8.2:** *Dropped fetlock secondary to flexor tendon damage*

## Puncture wounds

These wounds can be trouble. A small hole in the skin may be misleading when severe damage to deeper structures exists. It is always advisable that puncture wounds be examined and probed thoroughly by your veterinarian. Reason being is that an understanding of anatomy is paramount so that the safety of deeper structures, such as joints, can be assessed. Secondly, some punctures involve a projectile that may have broken off inside the wound. Careful probing to remove any foreign bodies is important.

Puncture wounds will typically not be sutured. They are left open so they can drain in the event that infection develops. Clean the surface of puncture wounds as described for lacerations. Bandage with a dry, clean dressing if possible. If you notice a puncture on the leg is draining a thick clear fluid, notify your veterinarian right away. There is a potential for joint or tendon involvement in these cases. Puncture wounds to the chest and abdomen are at risk of involving deeper structures as well. Puncture wounds to the foot will be described in the foot section of this chapter.

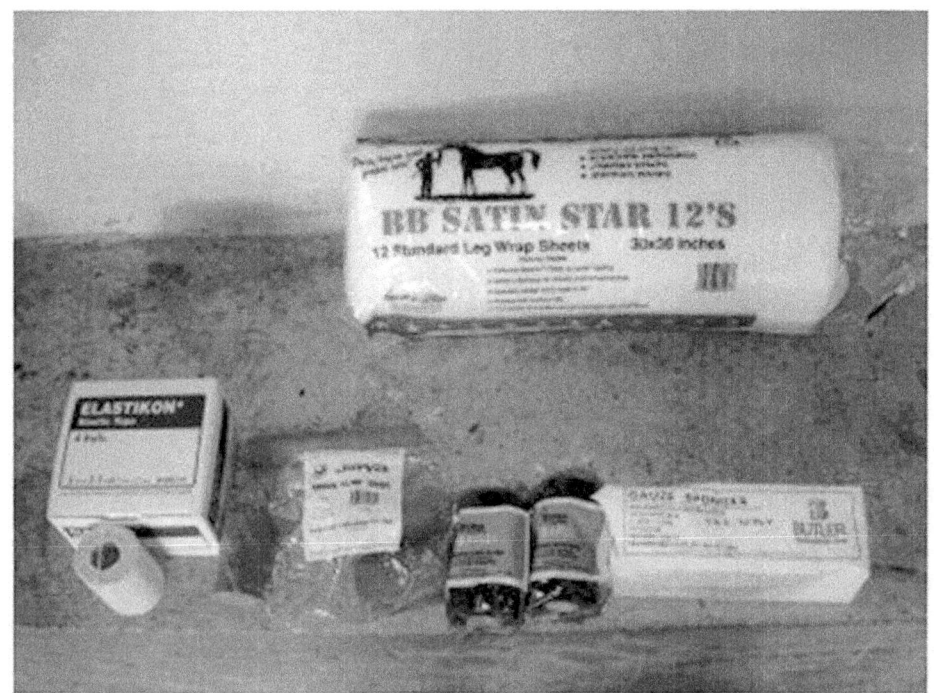

**Figure 8.3a:** *Bandage supply materials*

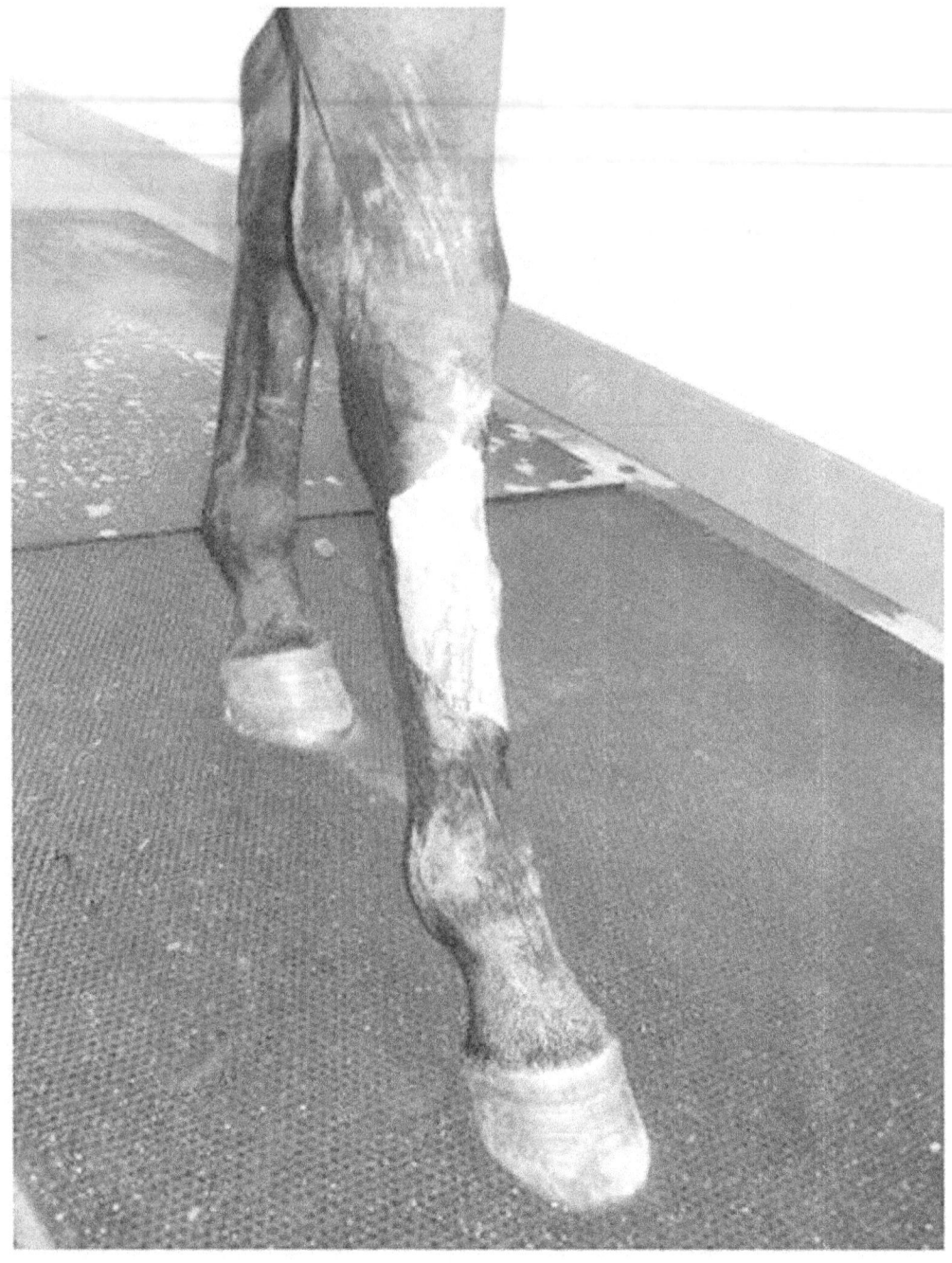

**Figure 8.3b:** *Wound cleaned before bandaging*

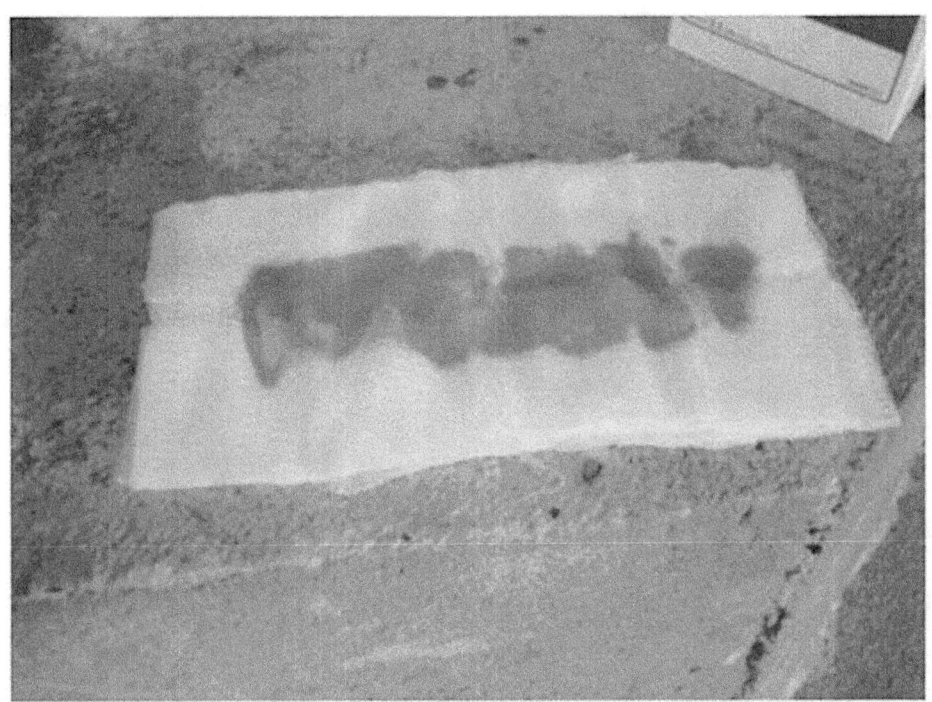

**Figure 8.3c:** *Primary dressing of 4x4s prepared with wound salve*

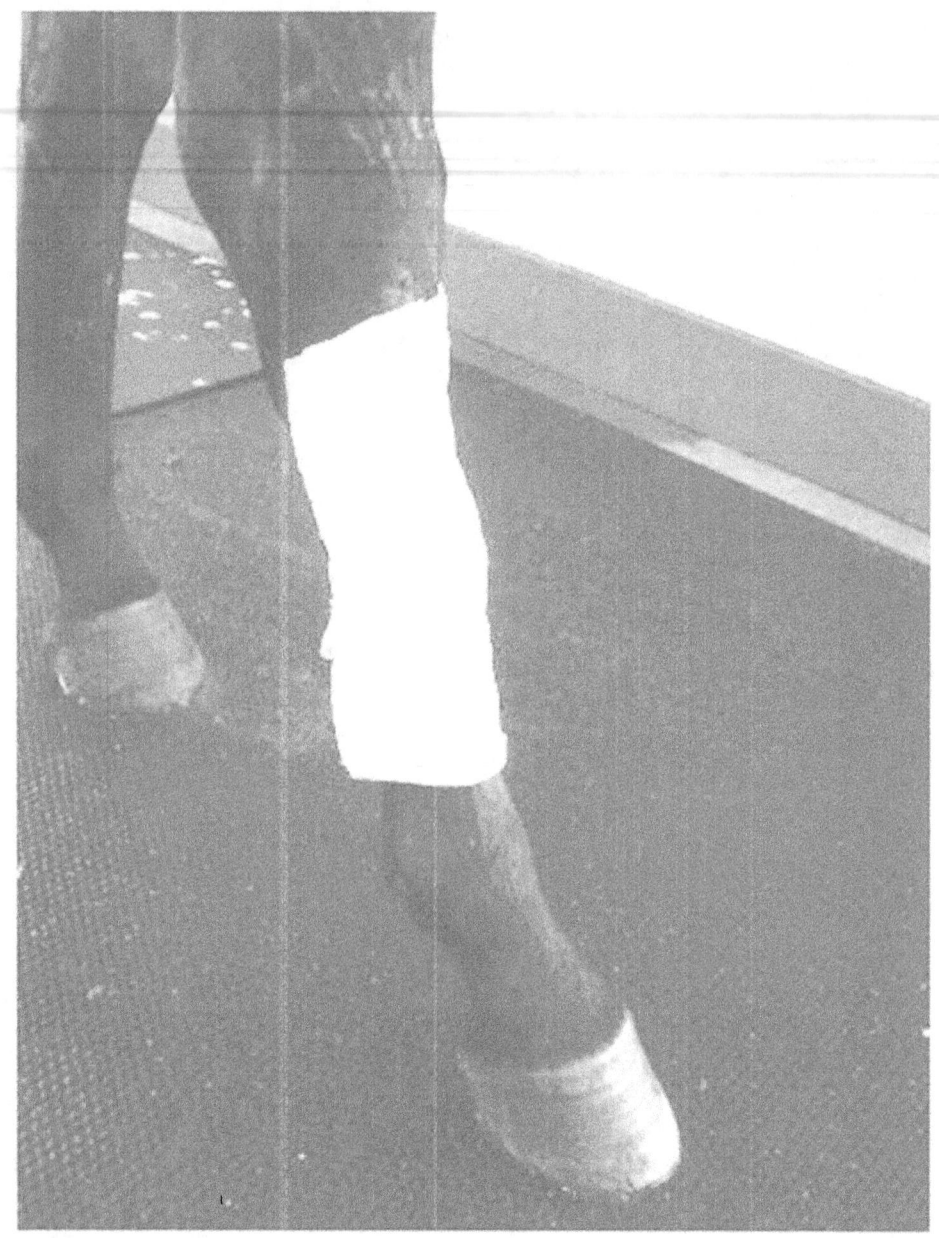

**Figure 8.3d:** *Dressing applied to leg*

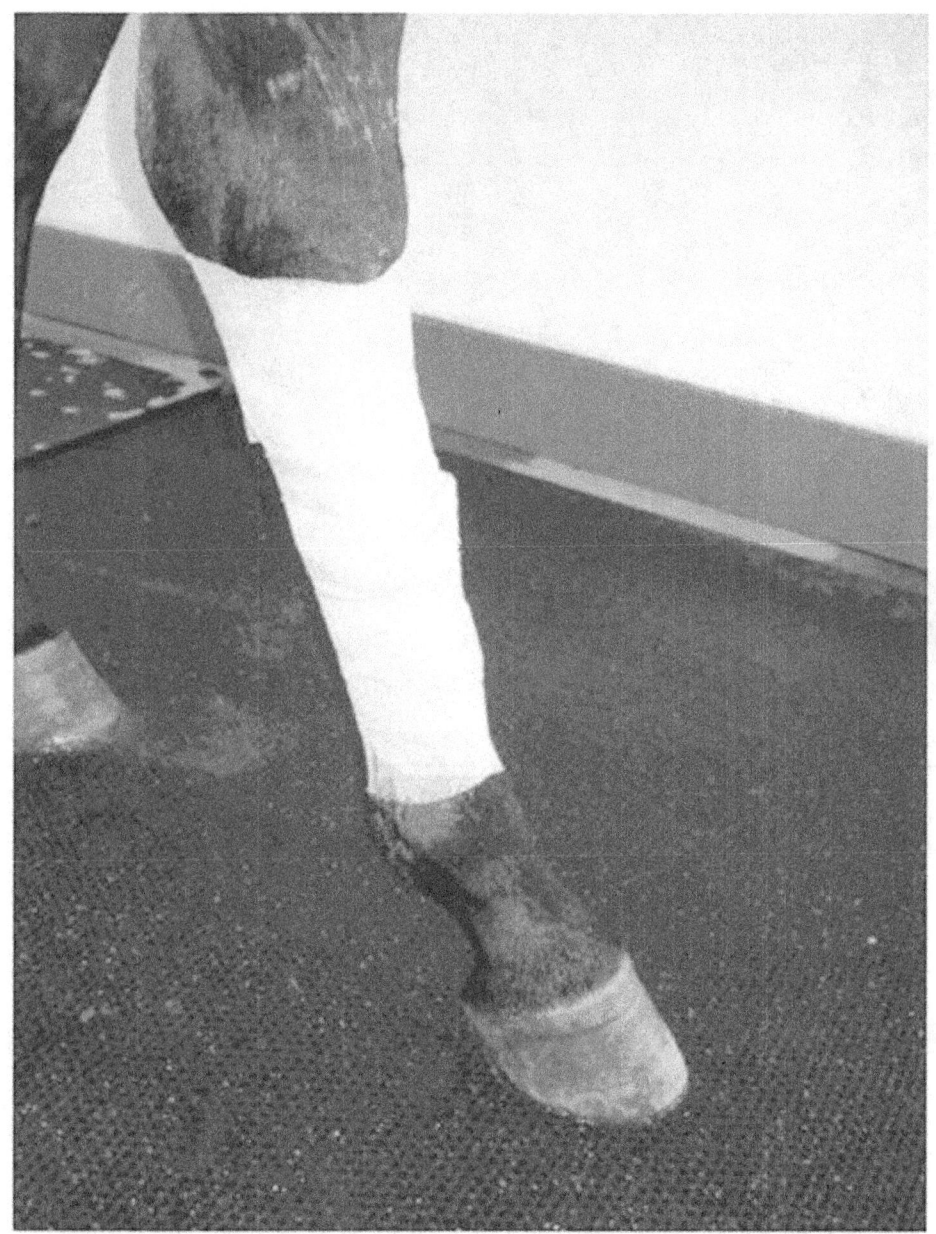
**Figure 8.3e:** *Dressing secured with 3inch roll brown gauze. Do not pull too tight*

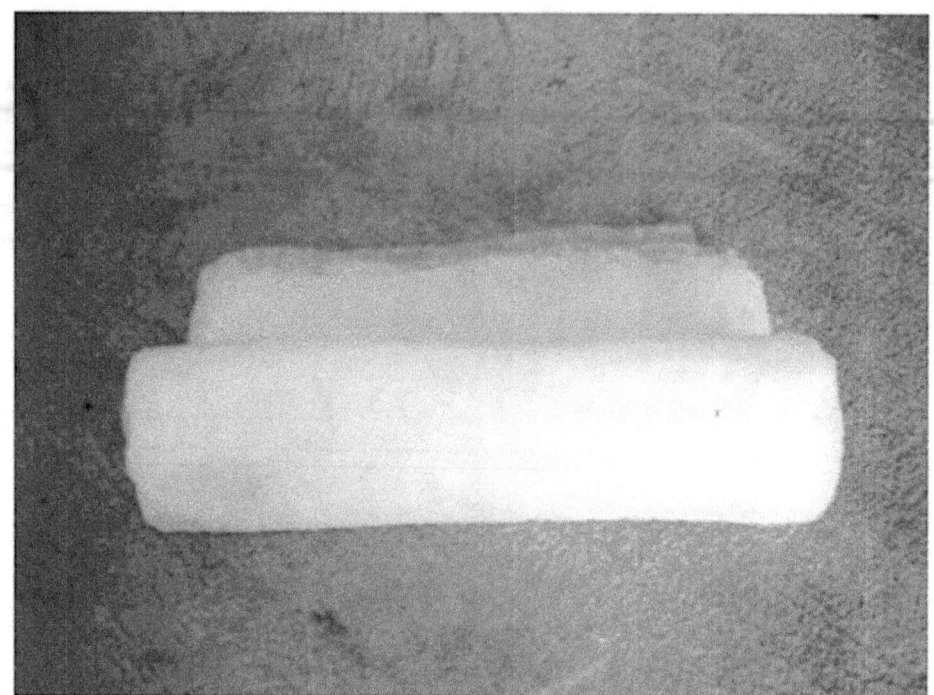

**Figure 8.3f:** *Sheet cotton rolled*

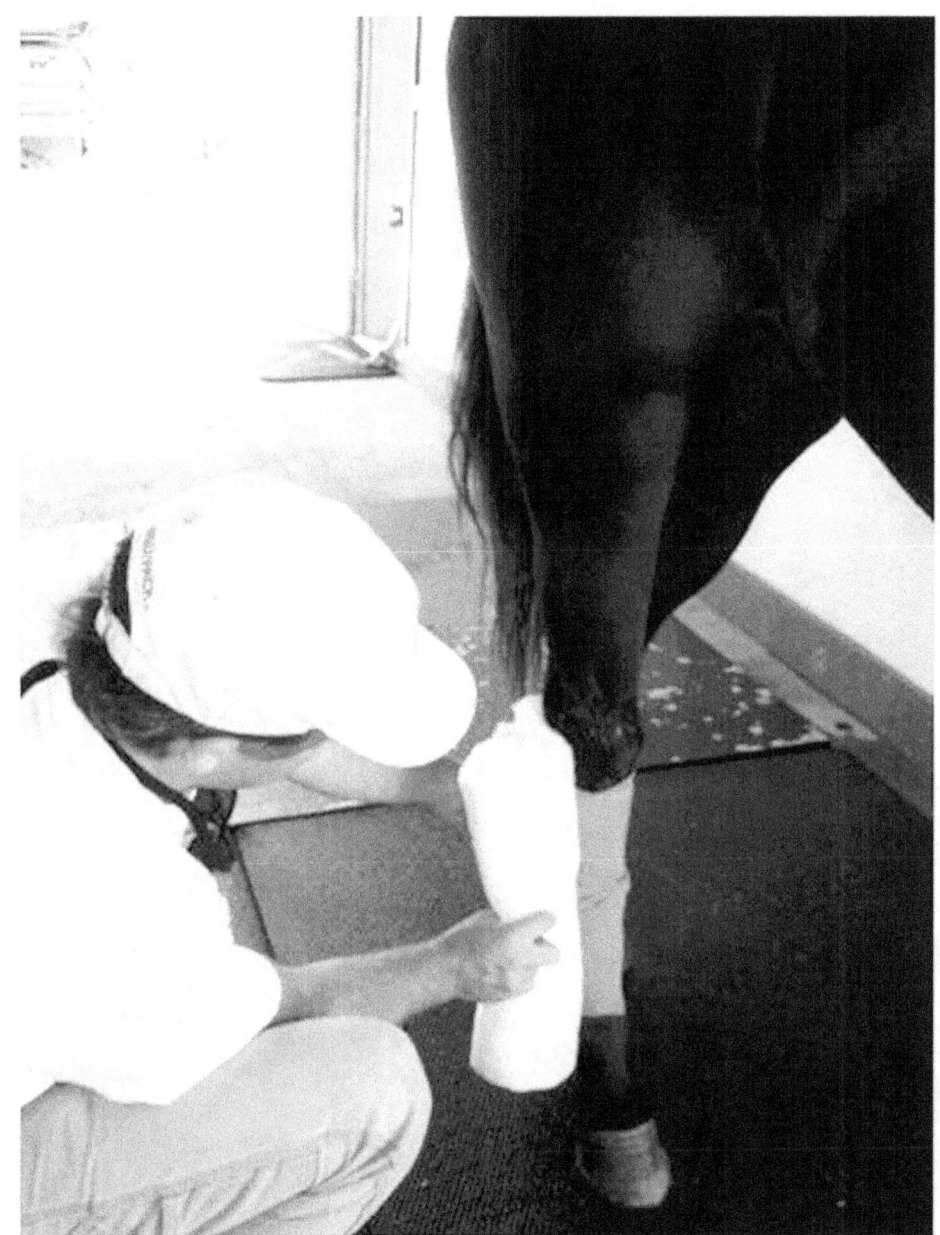

**Figure 8.3g:** *Applying sheet cotton over primary dressing*

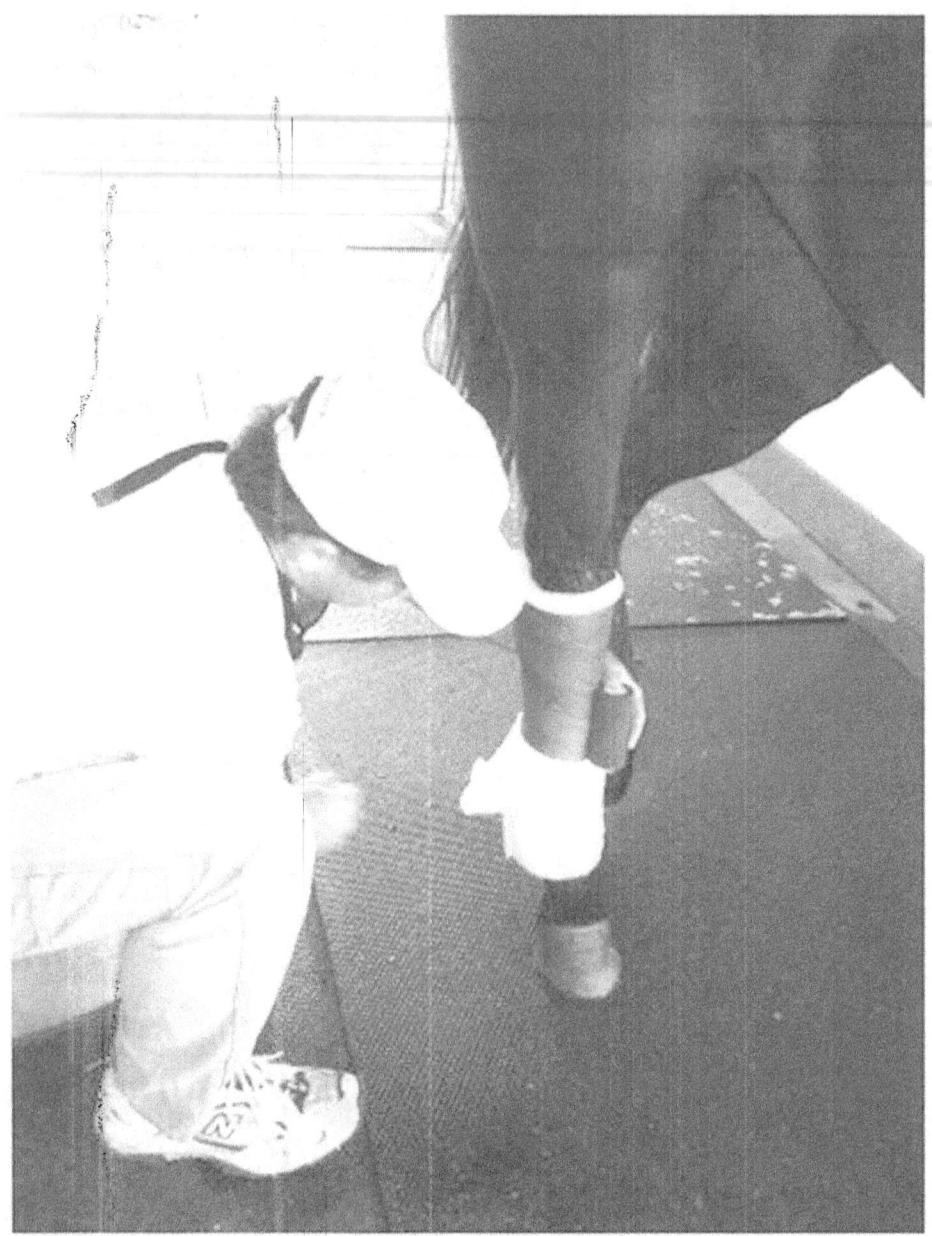

**Figure 8.3h:** *Securing sheet cotton with VetWrap*

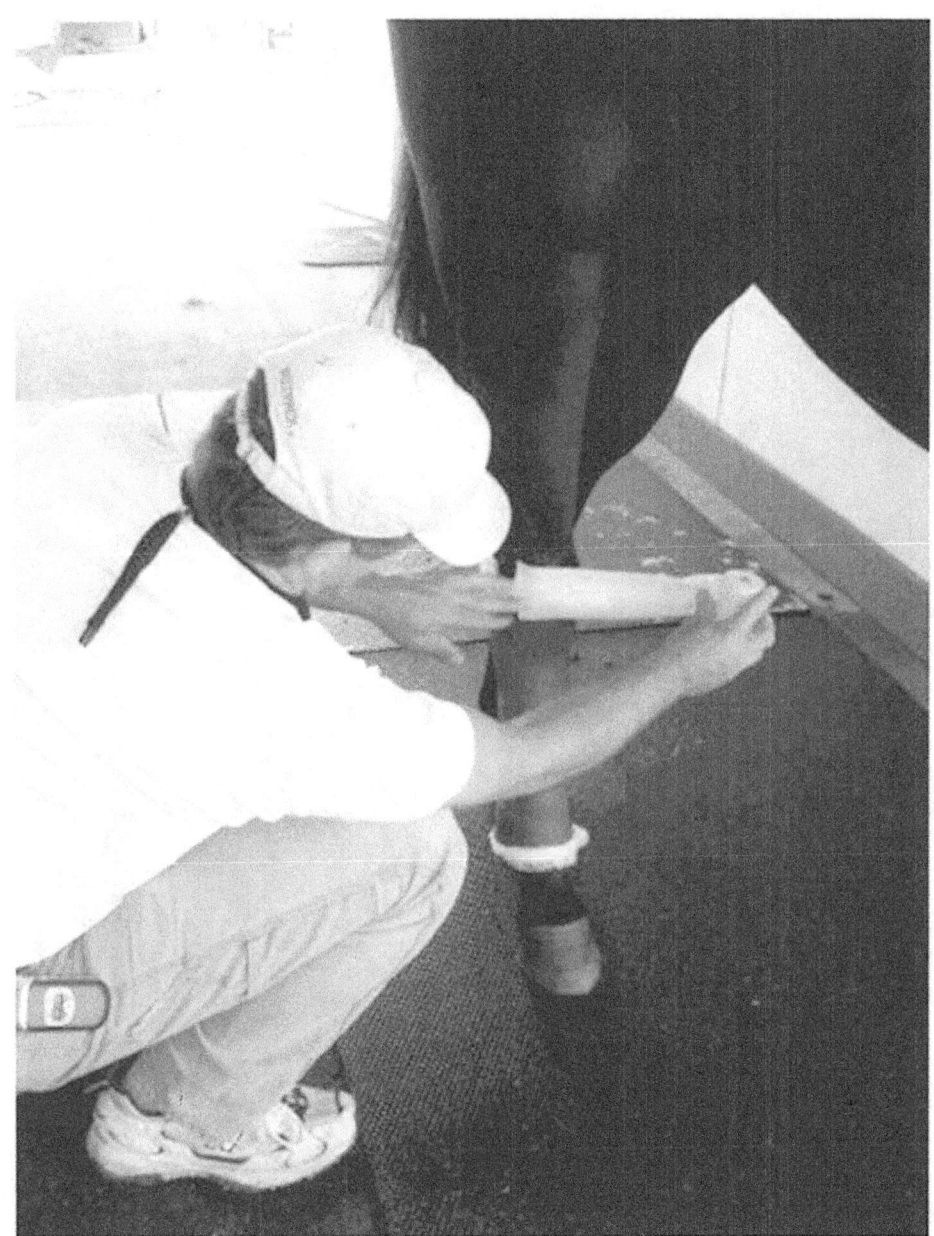

**Figure 8.3i:** *Elastikon applied to top edge of leg wrap*

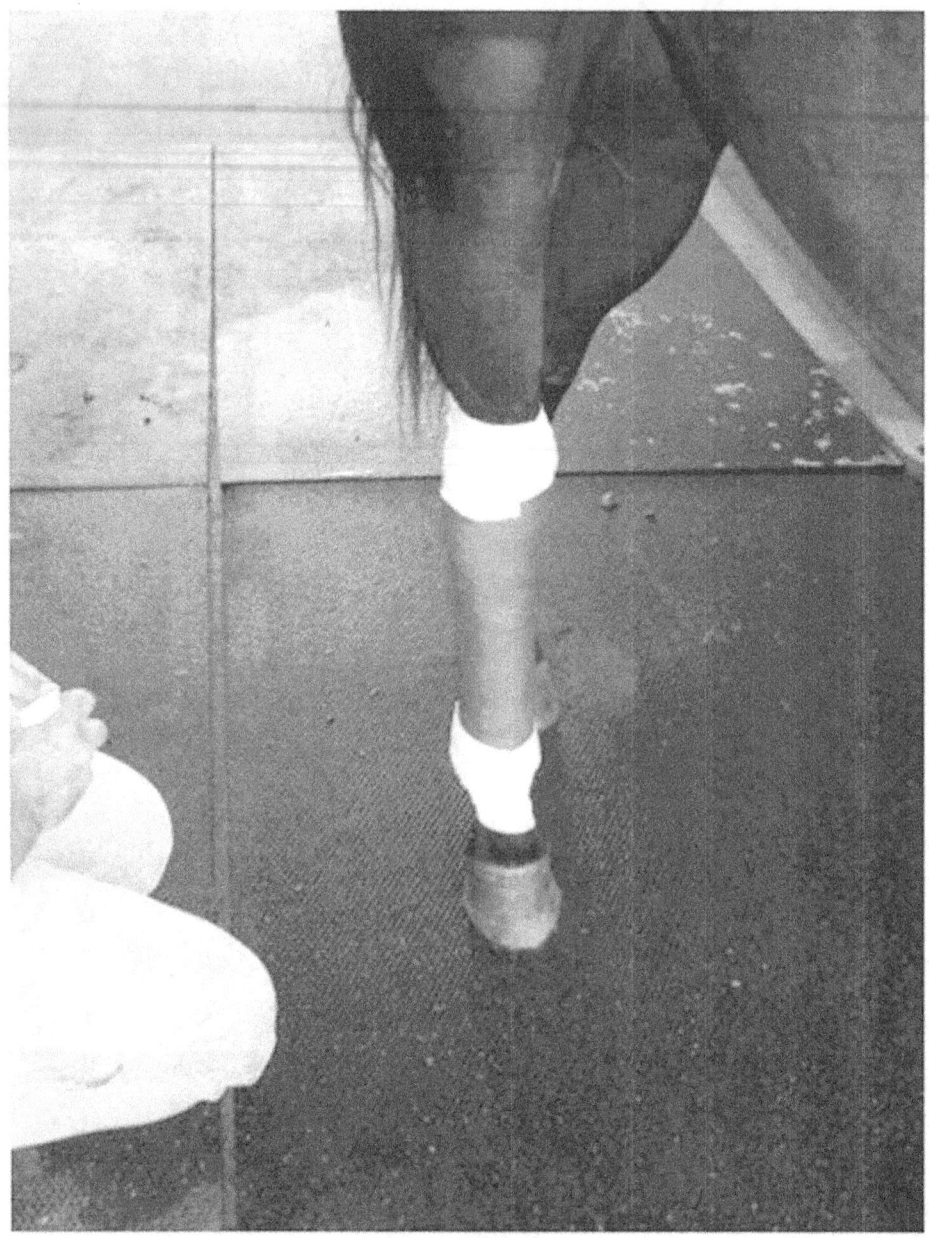

**Figure 8.3j:** *Elastikon to bottom edge of wrap*

# Infection

Any laceration or puncture wound can potentially develop infection. Generally these are superficial and do not pose much of a concern as long as the wound is cleaned and seems to be healing normally. If there seems to be excessive swelling, heat, drainage and/or foul odor there is likely infection present. If the infection has penetrated deeper in the tissue, more important underlying structures could be at risk.

Lacerations and/or punctures to the back side of the legs where the tendons are located should be closely examined to rule out tendon involvement. An infected tendon sheath could be the end of an athletic career or even terminal for the horse if infection is severe. Any puncture that is in close proximity to a joint should be thoroughly examined as well. Punctured joints may weep a clear to yellow fluid when initially injured. This is a red flag that action should be taken to prevent infection. As with infected tendon sheaths, infected joints could end a horse's career or his life!

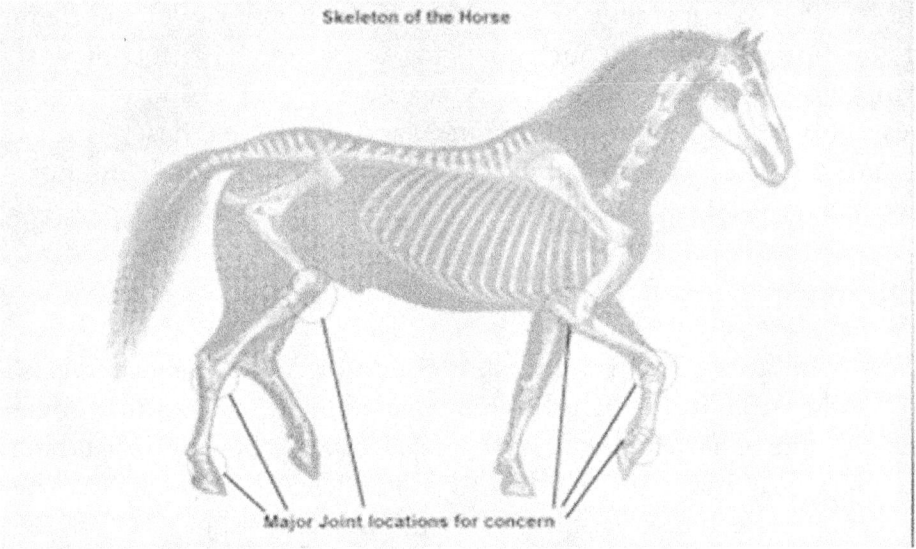

**Figure 8.4:** *Major joint locations*

# Burns

Burns can result from exposure to high heat as with a fire or from chemicals that are corrosive. Burns can be graded in severity as first, second, and third degree burns. In first degree burns, there is very superficial damage as with sunburn. Keep the horse in the shade and apply cool water, antibiotic, and aloe vera creams. Silver sulfadiazine, which usually requires a prescription, is an excellent antibiotic cream for burns.

Second degree burns are much more painful than first degree and can cause blistering. If the skin is blistered allow the blisters to remain a day or two before draining. This allows the underlying tissue to regenerate somewhat. At this time apply antibiotic creams. Pain relief can be helped with the use of phenylbutazone or flunixin meglumine, which are both available prescription only.

Third degree burns involve the full thickness of the skin. There is an added risk of shock and systemic infection that can accompany these burns. The management of the shock is paramount over the treatment of the burns. Assess your horse for any signs of impending shock. Symptoms of shock include high heart rate, cold clammy extremities, weak pulse, poor mucous membranes, and tremors. These burn victims require intensive care and will still have a very guarded prognosis for recovery.

# Hives

Hives is another name for a clinical condition known as urticaria. They are raised areas in the skin that may resemble an insect sting. Hives is a clinical sign of an allergic response. They may be few in numbers or hundreds may cover the whole body. The allergic response may be due to something eaten, a vaccine reaction, an insect sting, or exposure to a skin irritant. If the only sign is hives, you may be able to hose the horse with cool water and remove the offending source, if known. In many cases, the hives may disappear within 24 to 48 hours. If there is still no improvement within 24 hours, you may need to contact your veterinarian to obtain therapy to reduce the immune response.

## Acute leg swelling and cellulitis

Acute means that a condition or illness has occurred in a short period of time, such as overnight or within a day. Acute swelling(s) in the leg(s) should be examined thoroughly for any puncture or break in the skin. If so, refer to punctures and lacerations as described above. If the horse's temperature is normal and the horse is not in severe pain from the swelling and there is no apparent break in the skin, try hosing the leg first and then re-evaluate the horse in 12-24 hours. If improved, continue with the same therapy until better. If the swelling is accompanied by pain and lameness or fever, contact your veterinarian.

There may be a number of problems such as infection or tendon or joint injuries. It is important to determine the cause of the swelling so that the proper therapy is implemented. For instance, a tendon pull usually requires strict stall rest, whereas edema in the limb can benefit from turn out, and cellulitis requires antibiotic therapy. Acute leg swelling could be a clinical sign for certain viral diseases. If the horse is experiencing a fever and has swelling in all four legs, isolation is recommended.

## Venomous Bites

As mentioned in the respiratory chapter, venomous bites can pose an emergency situation. Typically, the lower extremities and the nose are involved with snake bites, but any part of the body could be affected by other insect or arthropod bites. If the horse is clinically stable after performing your physical exam, you can then concentrate on cleaning the bite area and take measures to reduce swelling. Cold hosing can be used in the earlier stages followed by warm and cold alternating after several hours.

Many venomous bites will cause the tissue around the bite area to die from the poisons in the venom. Therefore, there will be odor and drainage after the tissue begins to die. For this reason, antibiotic therapy is usually instituted, along with aggressive wound flushing to remove the decaying tissue. Some wounds may need to be lanced open to provide adequate drainage. Bandaging is often helpful in the lower limbs to provide support and keep the damaged area free of further contamination. If the horse is lame, the opposite limb should have a support wrap as well to help with the additional load bearing.

## Hematomas

Hematomas are soft, fluid-filled swellings that result from blunt trauma. The skin is usually not broken and there may be no pain associated with the swelling. A hematoma is formed when a blood vessel under the skin is ruptured and bleeds for a while before clotting. Hematomas tend to occur over thick, muscular areas such as the neck, chest, and buttocks. They can range in size from golf ball to volleyball sized.

If the hematoma is relatively small, it can be left alone. In most cases they will resorb back into the body with no after effects. Draining a small hematoma could potentially cause an unnecessary infection. Larger hematomas usually need to be drained and flushed to allow the skin to adhere back to the underlying tissues. It is common to administer an antibiotic during the healing process.

## Exuberant granulation tissue (Proud flesh)

Proud flesh is a unique phenomenon that occurs in horses more so than other species. In wounds of the lower legs that are left to heal without suturing, some degree of proud flesh will occur. In some cases, the tissue can be overwhelming and may need to be removed or trimmed back to allow proper granulation and contraction of the skin edges.

Proud flesh can be prevented or greatly reduced with the proper use of bandaging and some topical medications. There is a myriad of proud flesh preparations available, many from your personal veterinarian.

Some may be purchased over the counter. Discuss with your veterinarian what they believe to work best.

Much research has been devoted to equine wound management. Complete textbooks on wound management are available as well. Remember not to use these preparations on fresh wounds unless indicated. They are intended for wounds that are already granulating and have only superficial if any infection.

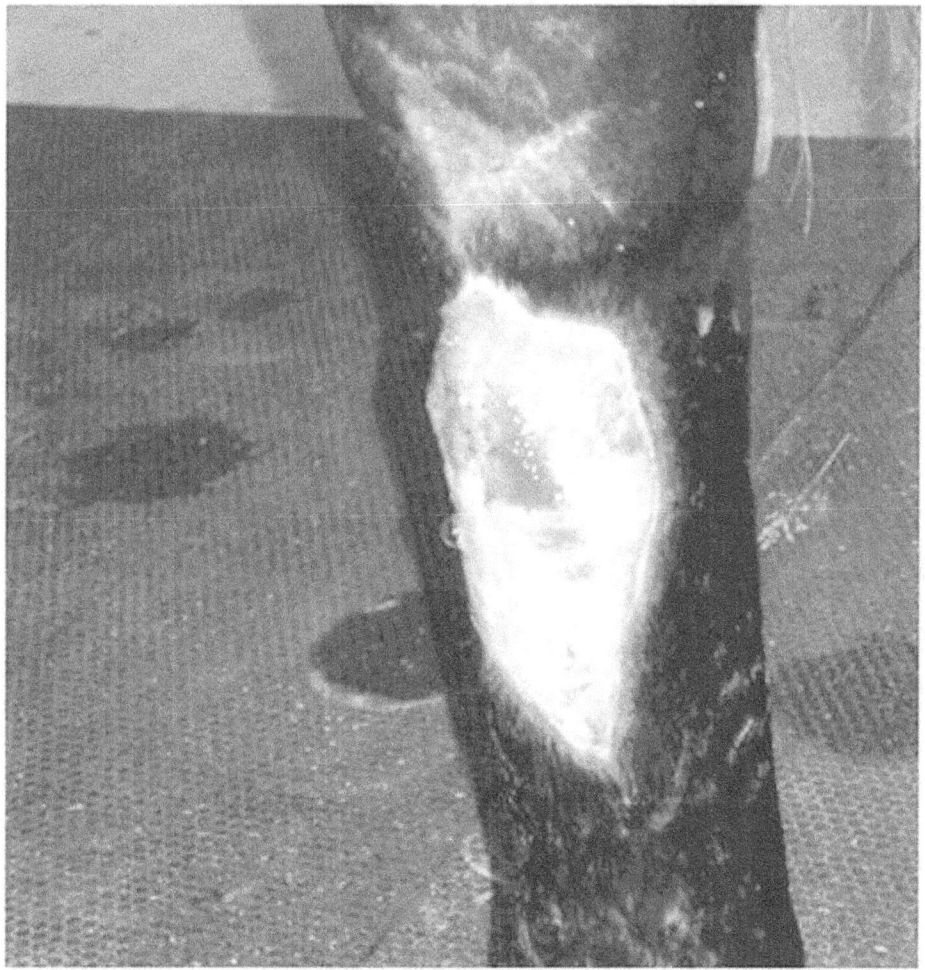

**Figure 8.5a:** *Granulating wound*

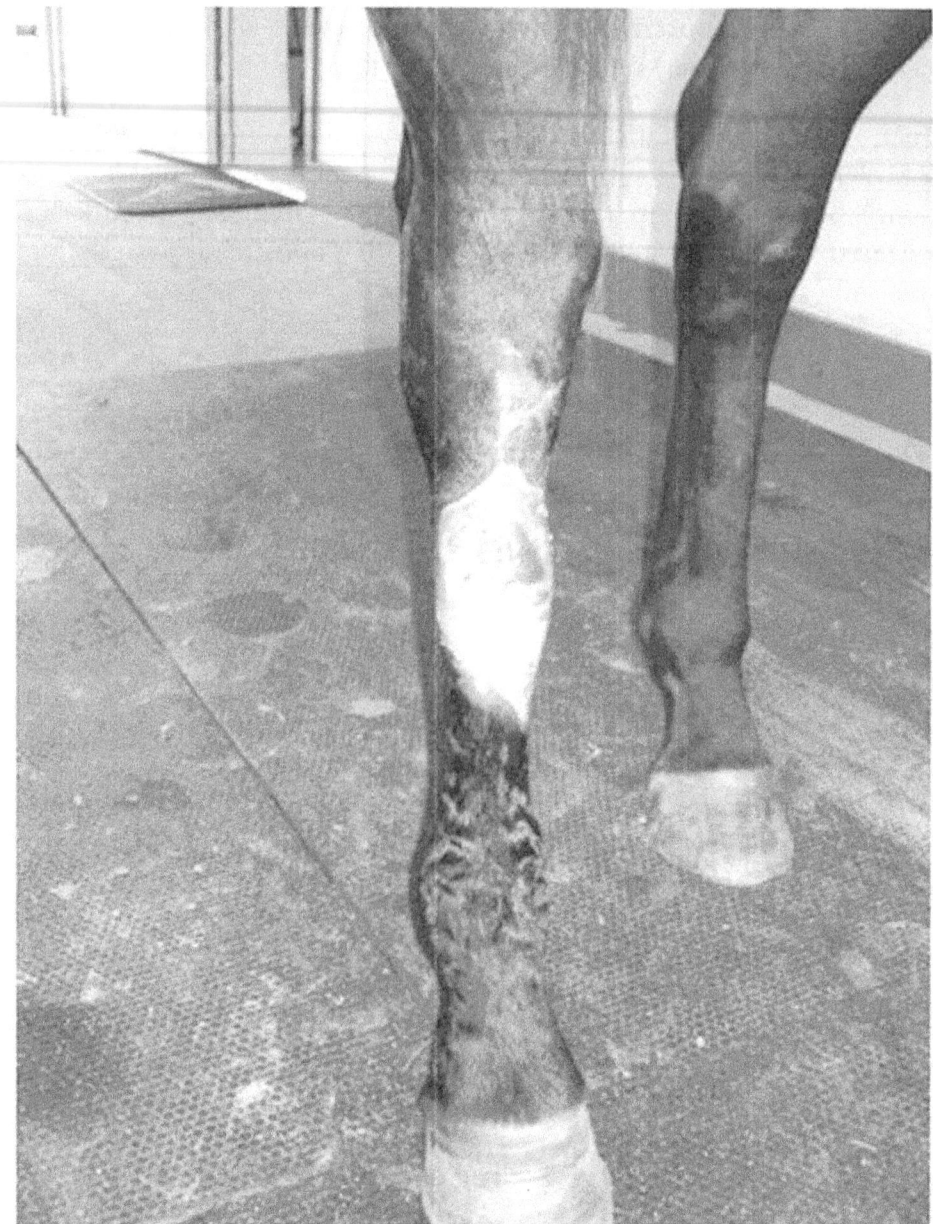

**Figure 8.5b:** *Granulation tissue*

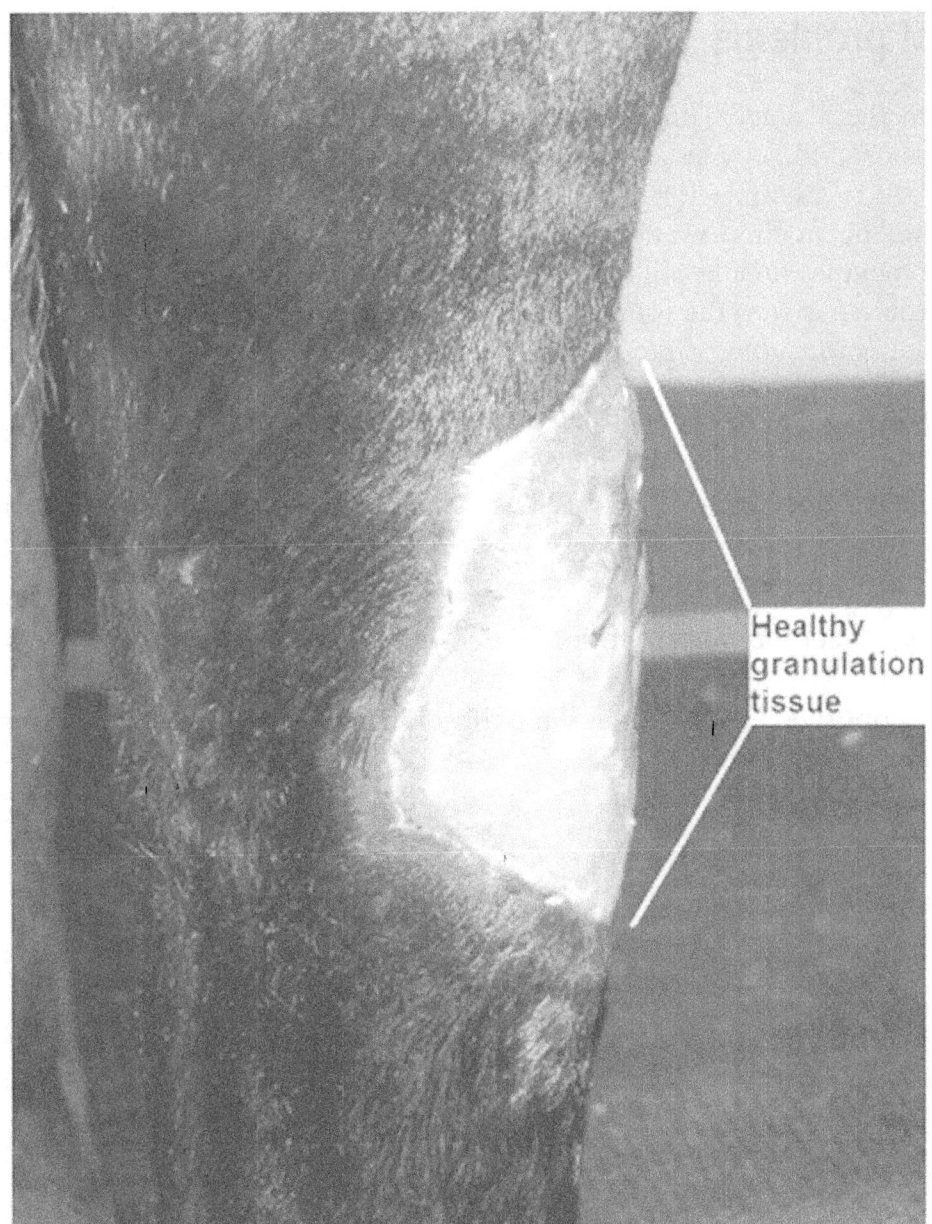

**Figure 8.5c:** *Healthy granulation tissue*

# Foot problems

On the average, lameness associated with the foot is very common as opposed to lameness elsewhere in the limb. The foot is always the first place to examine for acute lameness issues. Foot problems can cause swelling in the lower legs which can be misleading for many people. Sometimes people will tend to narrow in on the swelling when the actual problem is with the foot. Be prepared to perform an examination of the foot before going on to the rest of the limb.

## Hoof Exam

**Assess hoof heat**. Do this by feeling the affected limb's hoof, then feeling the normal limb's hoof for comparison. Any discrepancy could mean a problem in the warmer foot.

**Try to feel the pulses in the fetlock**. Cup your hand and gently assess the pulses behind the fetlocks as illustrated. Compare with the opposite limb. Bounding/throbbing pulses usually indicates a problem.

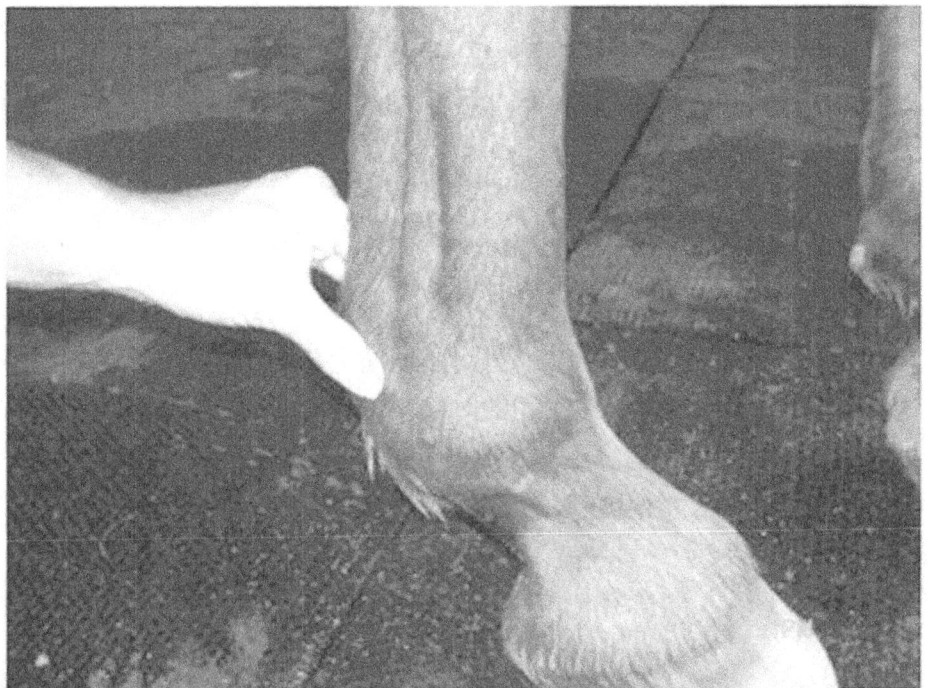

**Figure 8.6:** *Digital pulse evaluation*

- **Try tapping gently on the outside wall of the hoof**. Use something wooden or plastic such as a screwdriver handle. Remember not to whack the foot too hard! A gentle but firm tap that produces repeatable responses from the horse is all that is needed. Compare again with the opposite limb.

- **Apply pressure.** Apply point pressure with your fingertip around the whole coronary band. In many cases of unresolved hoof abscesses, there will be pain palpated in these areas due to impending abscess rupture.

- **Inspect the bottom/sole of the hoof**. Thoroughly pick and brush clean the surface. It may even be advantageous to use a bit of water to see the solar surface clearly. Inspect for cracks, bruises, punctures and foreign bodies. You may use the handle of the screwdriver again to tap or apply direct pressure over the sole to pinpoint a sore spot. Do not immediately remove any foreign objects that may be imbedded in

Foot problems

the hoof. If there is a risk that the foreign object may be driven deeper in to the hoof, then it may be best to remove the object and note the exact location of penetration. Instead, call your vet, who may wish to x-ray the foot first with the foreign object in place, so that potential damage to deeper structures can be seen.

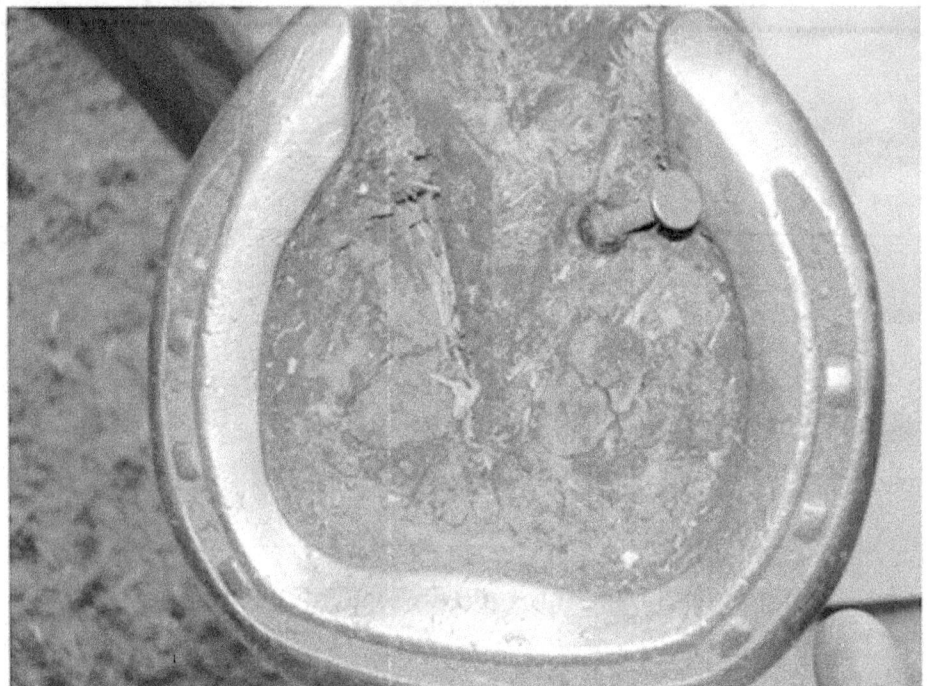

**Figure 8.7:** *Nail Imbedded in Frog Sulcus*

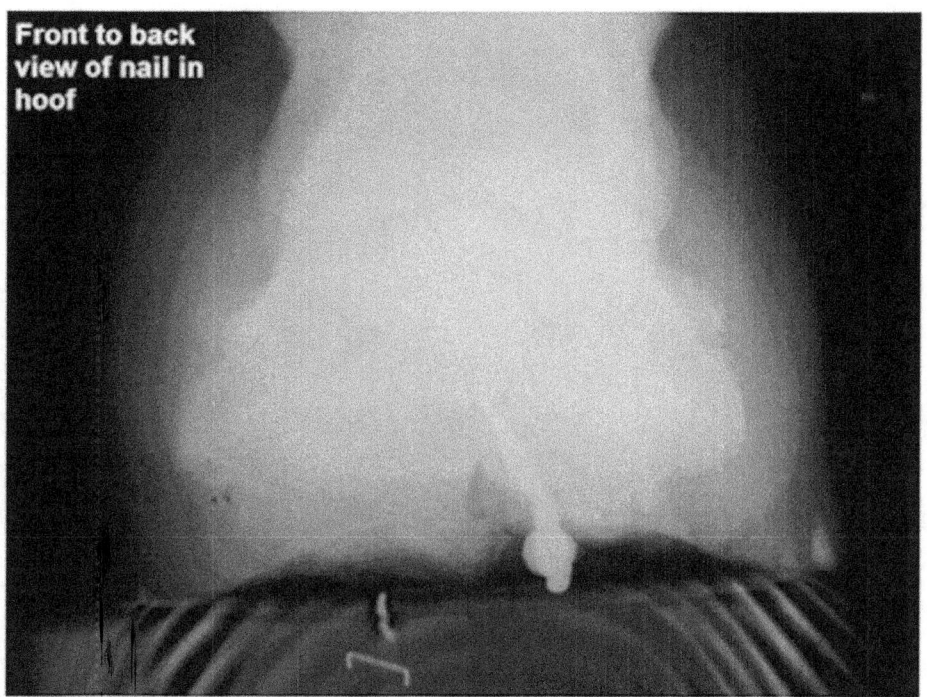

**Figure 8.7a:** *Front to Back X-ray of Nail in Hoof*

Foot problems

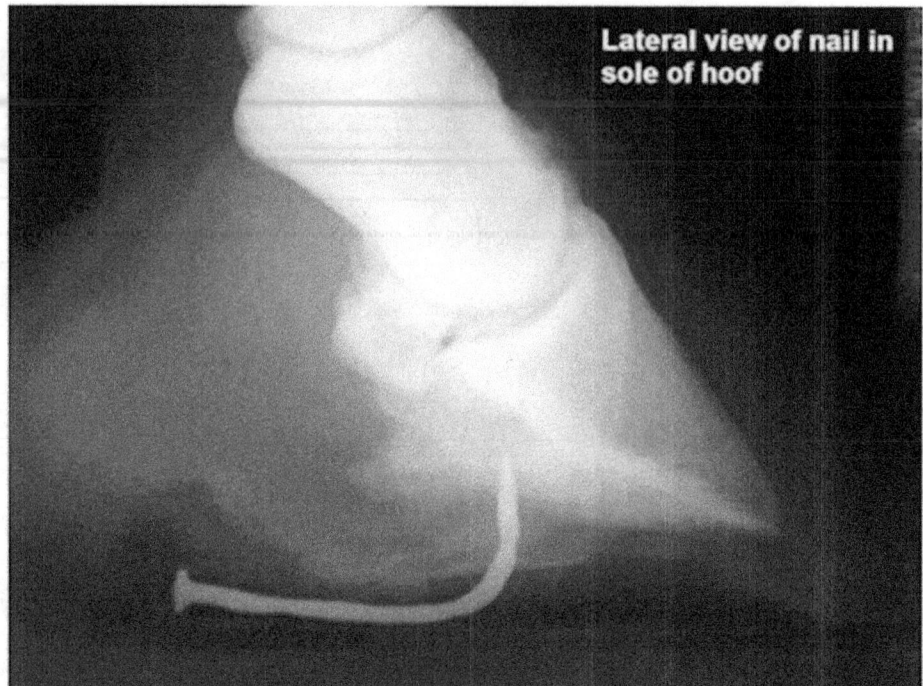

**Figure 8.7b:** *Lateral X-ray of Nail in Hoof*

**Remove shoe**. Be prepared to know how to remove a shoe if needed. Have your farrier or veterinarian instruct you on the tools needed and procedure to do this.

## Emergencies of the foot

Obviously not all conditions of the foot are emergencies. Punctures, foreign objects, and severe cracks can be cause for emergency attention. Sudden non-weight bearing with no apparent swelling in the limb could be a fractured coffin bone. Laminitis, which usually involves both front feet, is a valid emergency. Performing your exam and discussing your findings with your veterinarian can normally be enough information to deem the situation an emergency or not.

## Laminitis

Laminitis is defined as inflammation of the lamina, which is the tissue that essentially connects the outer hoof to the bone in the foot. It is helpful to view an illustration of this area in the foot.

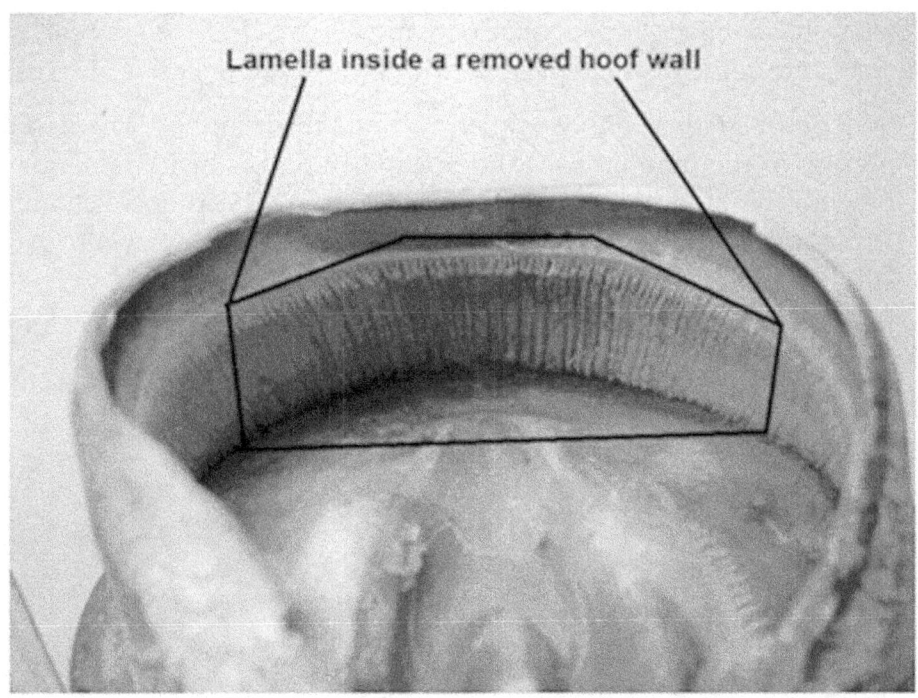

**Figure 8.8:** *Inside view of hoof wall depicting lamella*

Laminitis is among the most dreaded of all equine ailments. If anyone followed Barbaro's treatment after his race injury, you will have learned something about laminitis. Since laminitis treatment is such a huge aspect in equine health care, some equine veterinarians become specialized in the area and devote their whole practice to treatment of horses with foot problems. They are experts in their field and can provide the latest in treatment strategies and phenomenal care. In some of the most hopeless cases these veterinarians can salvage a treasured horse from euthanasia.

Prompt, immediate treatment is fundamental for the best outcome in laminitis cases. Know the clinical signs for laminitis. There are different forms of laminitis based upon the progression of the disease. Sometimes there is a predisposing factor that is known to initiate a spell of laminitis, sometimes the cause is unknown. We will list some of the more common triggers. Regardless of the cause or type of laminitis present, in an emergency situation you will treat all the same. The following are some of the typical but not always present clinical signs:

- Sudden or gradual onset of pain in both front limbs. This is rarely present in the hind limbs. The posture of a horse with laminitis will be with the hind limbs positioned far forward from normal, and the front limbs extended far forward as well. The horse may also have a stiff and stilted gait and be reluctant to turn.

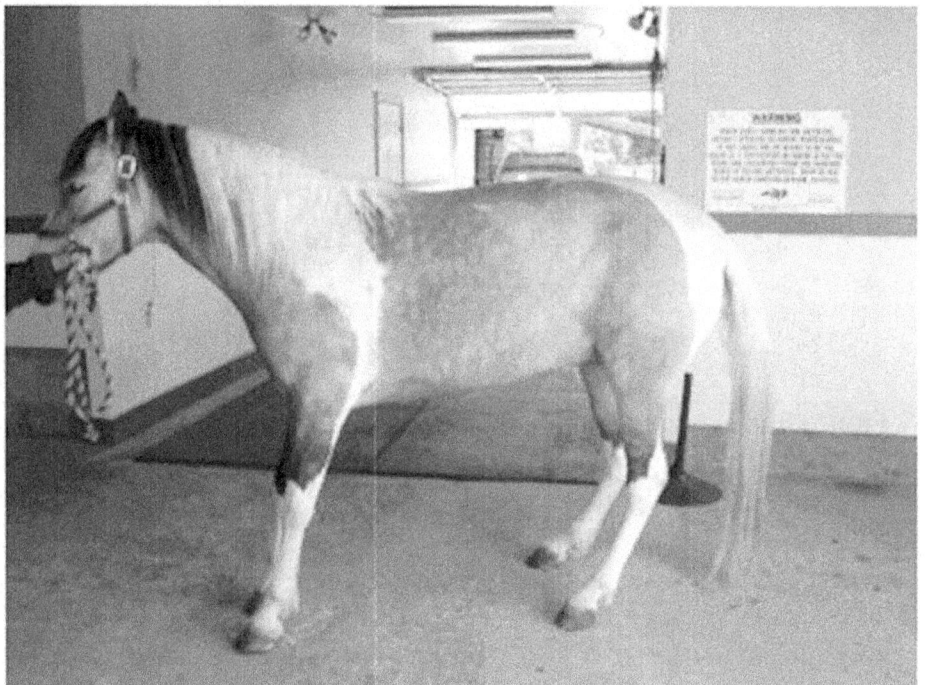

**Figure 8.9:** *Laminitis stance*

- Increased heat in the hooves and increased digital pulses in the fetlocks.

- Increased respiration and heart rate from severe pain.
- Constant shifting of weight in affected limbs.
- Variable increases in hoof temperature.
- Increase in the digital pulses. These are palpated just behind the fetlock.
- Increased heart and respiration rate due to pain.

Anything that causes a compromise to the blood flow of the lamina deep in the hoof can initiate an episode of laminitis. Certain diseases release toxins into the bloodstream that cause the smaller capillaries down in the foot to contract, thus causing a loss in oxygen, referred to as hypoxia, resulting in instability, inflammation, and subsequent deterioration of the laminar connection. Here is a list of some factors that could predispose the horse to laminitis:

- **Grain Overload**. As covered in more detail in the chapter on colic, grain or carbohydrate overload can alter the normal gut flora allowing the toxic bacteria to release harmful toxins that enter the bloodstream and cause vascular damage in the hoof.
- **Colic**. Many forms of strangulating colic can also release toxic principles into the bloodstream that will have an effect on the blood flow in the hoof.
- **Concussion to hoof**. Running on a hard surface, such as pavement, for extended periods of time can initiate laminitis.
- **Disease.** Any disease that causes endotoxemia or bacterial poisoning of the blood can initiate laminitis. Retained placentas and some plant toxins are known to cause endotoxemia. Potomac Horse Fever is linked with laminitis in many cases.
- **Prolonged weight bearing.** Prolonged weight bearing on one foot can initiate laminitis. If a horse sustains injury to a limb and does not return to even or close to even weight bearing within 10-14 days, the limb supporting most or all of the weight can be predisposed to laminitis.

## Treatment Plans for Laminitis

Obviously, as with many other diseases, prevention is the best treatment. If you can prevent the predisposing factors you can prevent laminitis in many cases. If however, you are dealing with an acute case of laminitis, you should be prepared to provide immediate therapy before mechanical breakdown occurs.

Medically, the horses are given appropriate anti-inflammatory drugs to decrease pain and swelling in the lamina. Corticosteroid anti-inflammatory medication such as dexamethasone should never be used. Other agents that may dilate blood vessels and improve blood flow can be initiated. If there is suspected infection, appropriate antibiotic therapy is initiated.

Mechanical treatment of the foot is paramount in conjunction with the medical therapies. Sole support is important to reduce further damage to the sensitive laminae. This can be performed initially with Styrofoam. The stall should be bedded deeply with shavings especially if the horse is staying down. Sand can also be used to provide support. Shoes should carefully be removed. Your veterinarian may elect to radiograph the feet with contrast dyes in the blood vessels to assess areas of low to no blood flow.

Radiographs are extremely important to characterize the coffin bone inside the hoof wall. Measurements of coffin bone position in the radiographs can be taken to determine underlying hoof problems that need to be addressed early in the treatment scheme. As mentioned earlier, specialty shoes can be used to reduce the tendon pull on the coffin bone, as well as enhance breakover in the foot. Breakover is usually at the tip of the toe in most horses. By pushing this point further back, it reduces the fulcrum effect that is negatively working to separate the hoof from the coffin bone.

To conclude, horses with laminitis should not be transported for long distances unless they have good sole support. If transport is necessary, such as to a treatment facility, discuss sole support techniques with the veterinarian in charge of therapy.

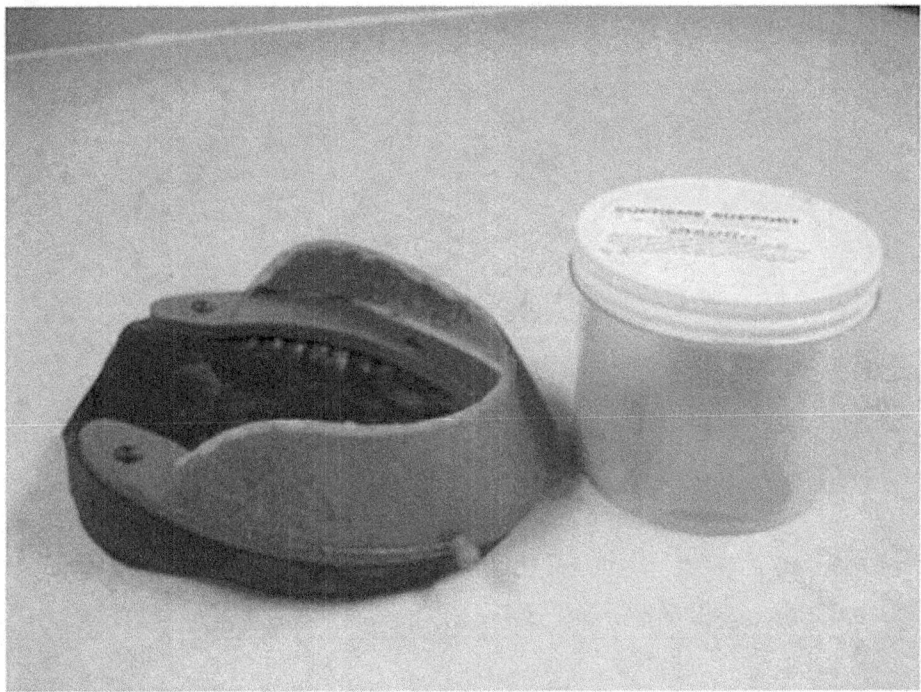

**Figure 8.10a:** *Example of commercially available support shoe and sole support*

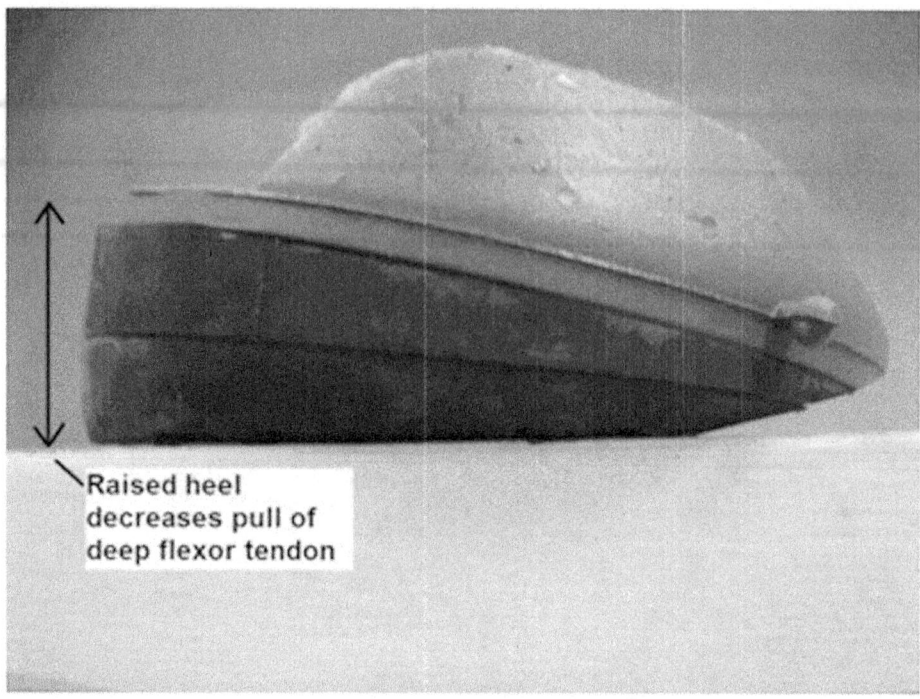

**Figure 8.10b:** *Support shoe side view*

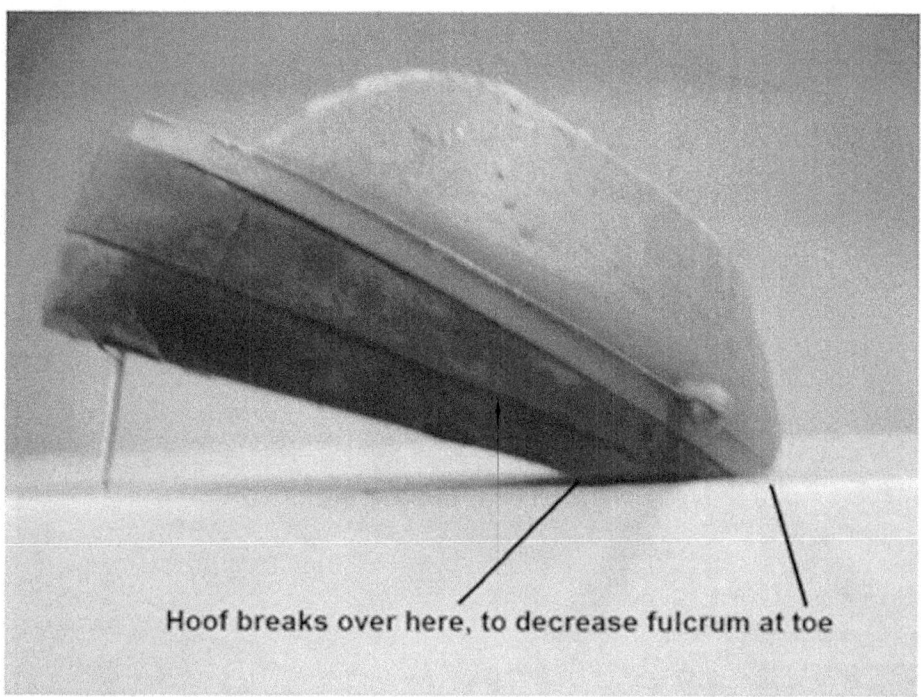

**Figure 8.10c:** *Support shoe depicting easier breakover when walking*

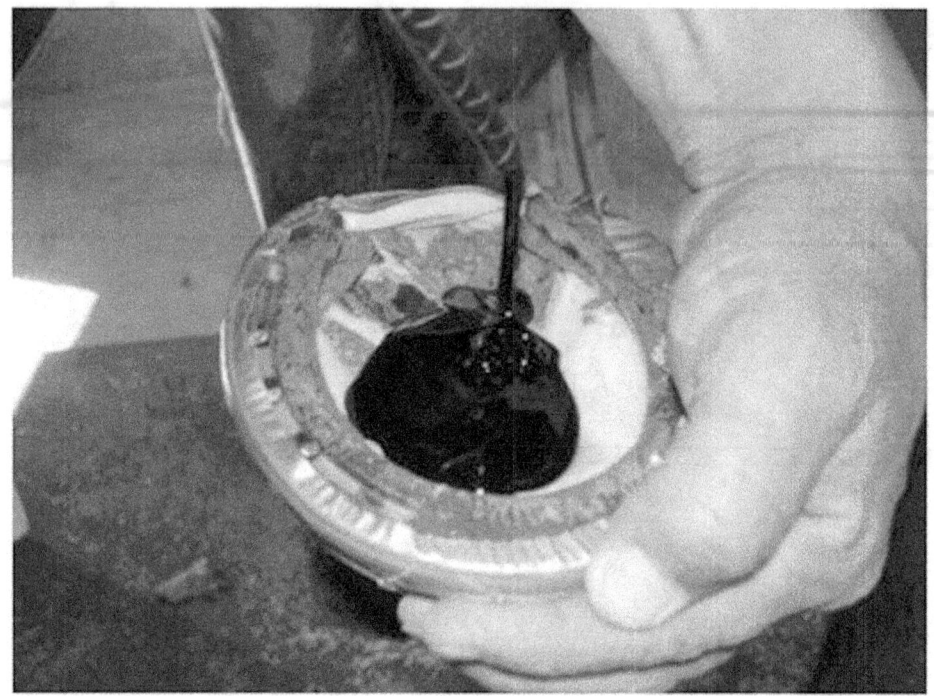

**Figure 8.10d:** *Pour-in support pad that creates perfect mold of foot for great support*

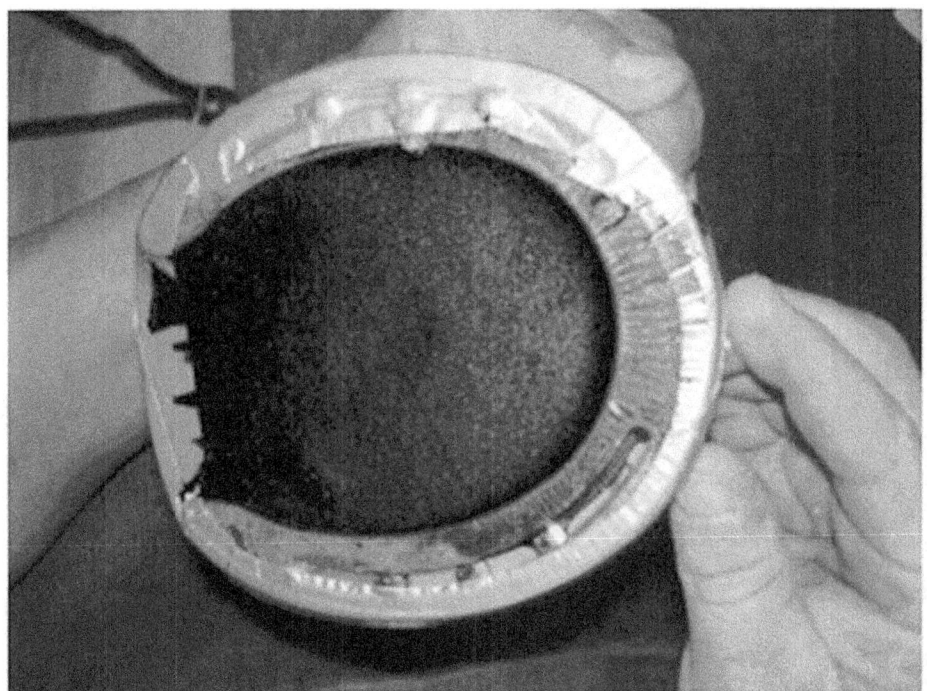

**Figure 8.10e:** *Pour-in pad after setting up*

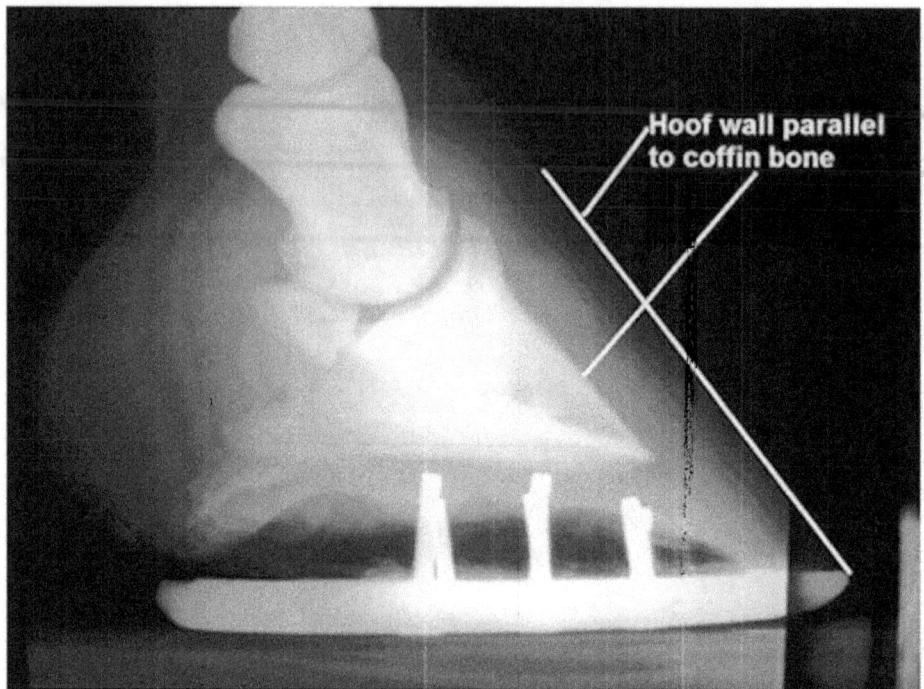

**Figure 8.11a:** *Normal hoof radiograph*

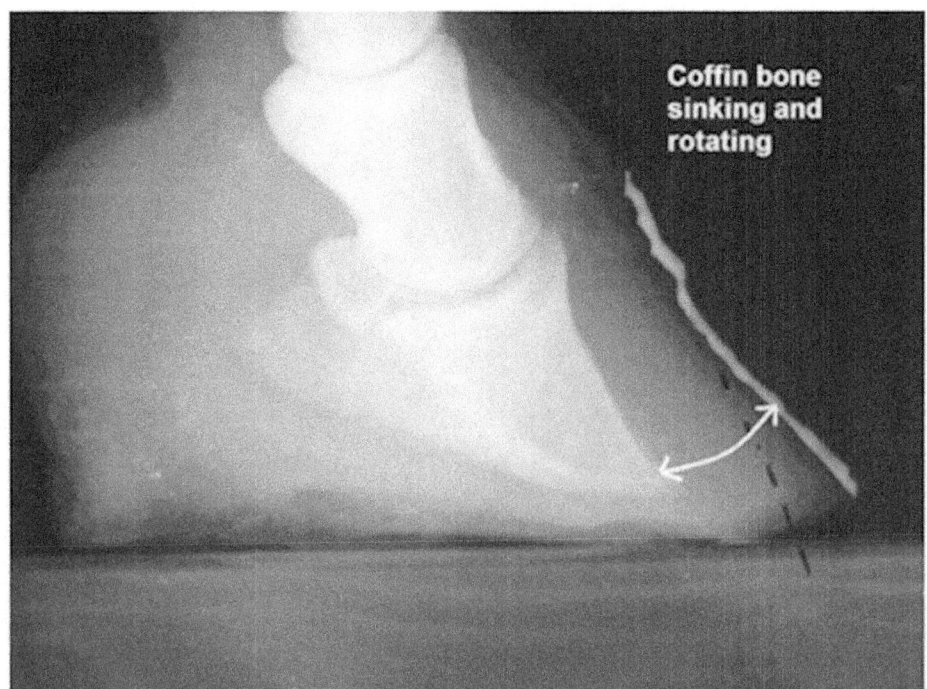

**Figure 8.11b:** *Radiograph of hoof with laminitis*

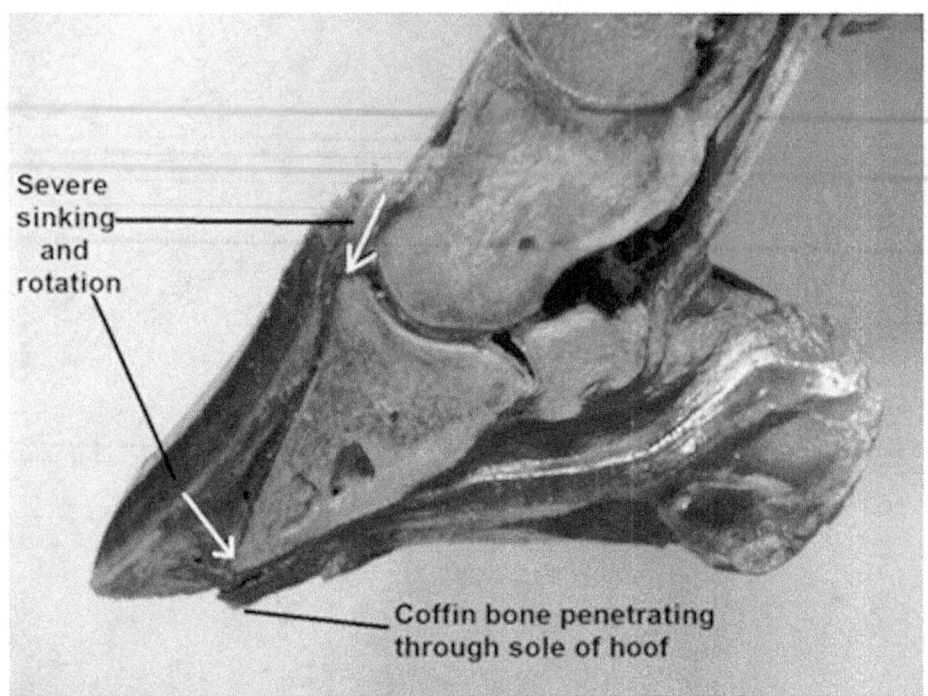

**Figure 8.11c:** *A chronic foundered hoof specimen*

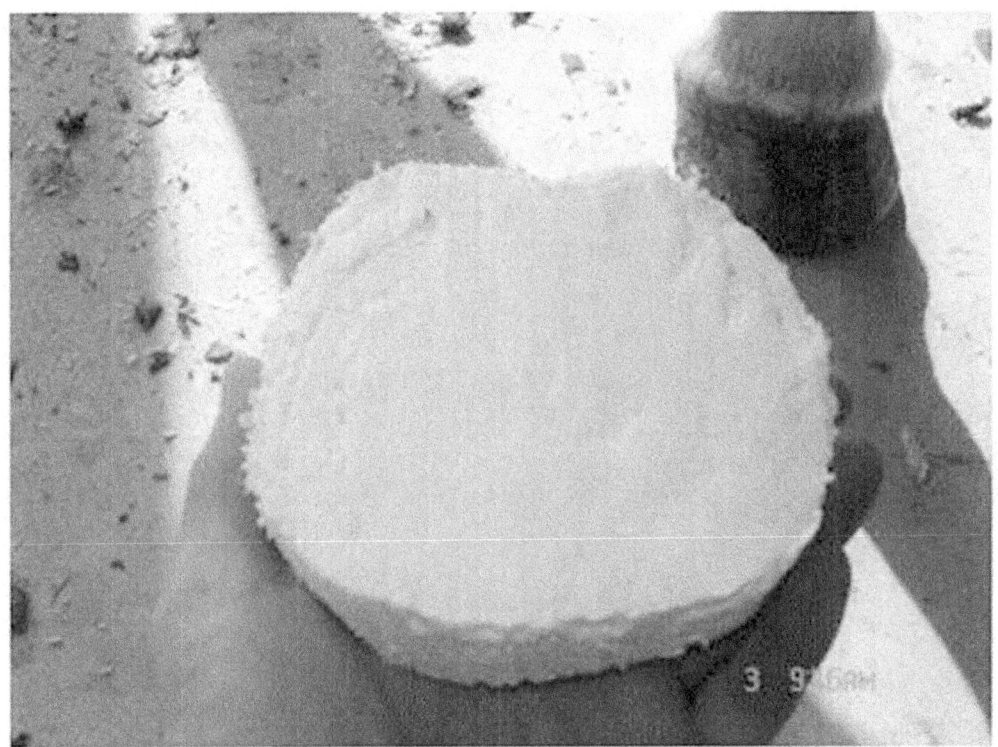

**Figure 8.12a:** *Styrofoam pad cut to hoof shape*

Foot problems

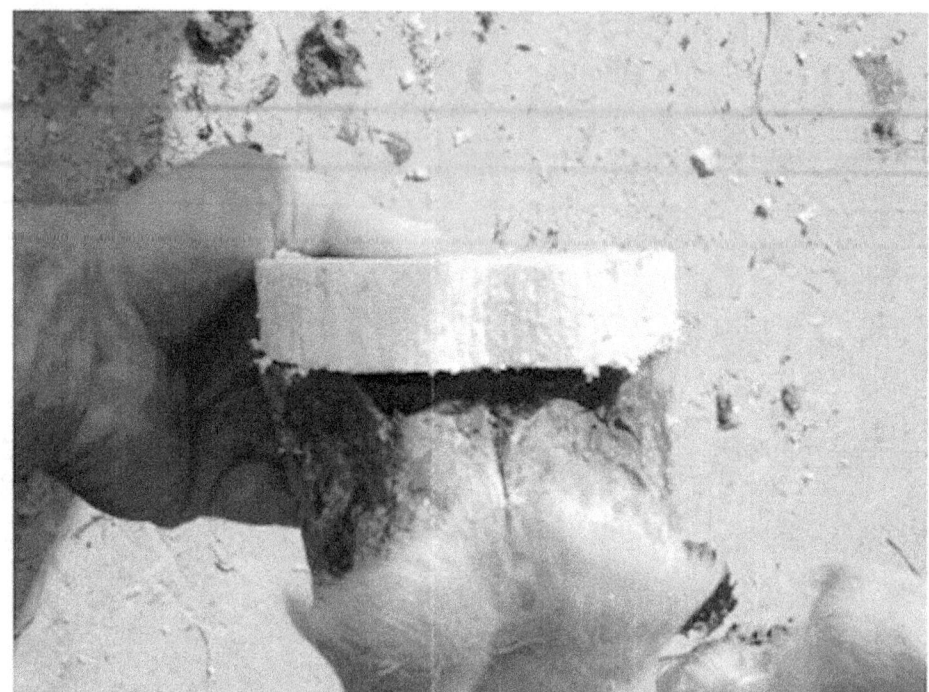

**Figure 8.12b:** *Foam pad applied to sole of hoof*

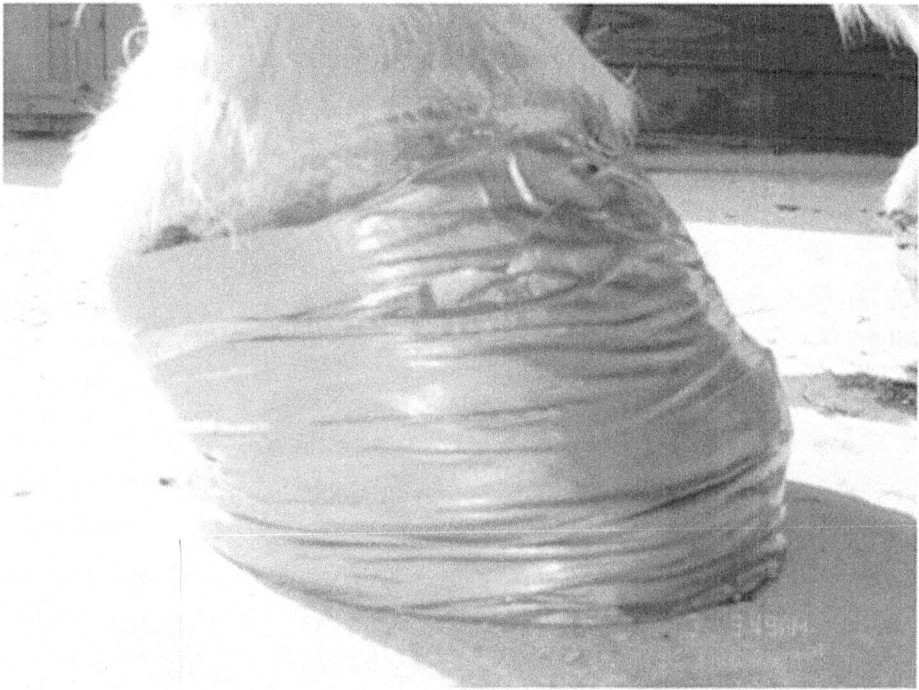

**Figure 8.12c:** *Foam pad taped to hoof*

In summary laminitis is among one of the toughest of equine diseases to treat. Much research has been devoted to why horses develop laminitis and how to effectively treat the disease both medically and mechanically. As with most disease processes, early detection and stabilization is paramount with laminitis. Do your research to ensure that all is being done to help your horse. Treatment can be rewarding but comes with a cost. Treating laminitis can be expensive and very time consuming. Be prepared for what may be a long battle toward recovery if your horse faces laminitis.

## Hoof Punctures

Punctures to the sole of the foot are relatively common. If you have ever had a new roofing job done on your barn, be sure to invest some money in a high powered rolling magnet to pick up any stray nails on the ground. Not all hoof punctures occur due to nails or metallic objects.

Wooden objects and glass are other sources that can penetrate the sole and cause damage. Regardless of the object, the site of puncture and depth of puncture is critical to the overall prognosis for recovery.

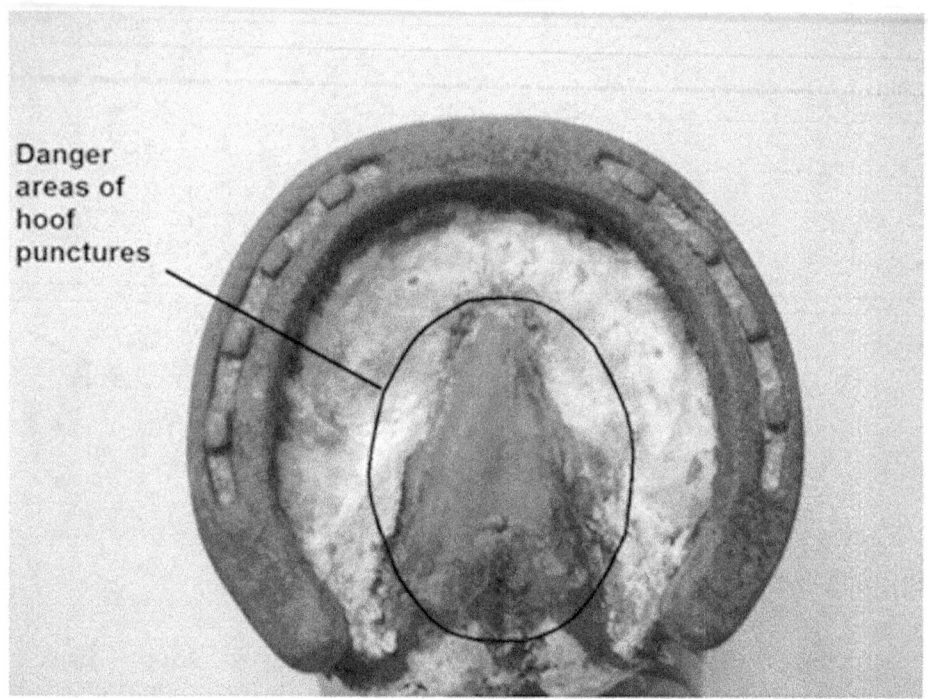

**Figure 8.13:** *Major areas of concern for hoof punctures*

The most obvious sign with foot punctures is of course lameness. Some horses may exhibit distal limb swelling and heat. If a foreign object is found during your exam of the foot, do not immediately remove it. Your veterinarian may elect to radiograph the foot with the foreign object in place to determine depth of penetration.

If there is potential for the object to be driven deeper into the foot, then thoroughly clean the area, and remove the object noting the depth and direction the object entered the foot. Be prepared to immediately bandage the foot before placing the foot back down. Perform this procedure on a concrete floor or use plywood or other materials in case the horse pulls the foot away during treatment.

Puncture wounds to the foot have a greater tendency for infection than other punctures elsewhere on the body since the foot is in constant contact with urine, feces, and other contaminates. Aggressive treatment by debriding or cutting away the hoof at the site of puncture and applying antibiotics directly to the area is routine. Heavy duty bandages, hoof boots, or special hospital plate shoes are used during the treatment period. Systemic antibiotics may be used in some cases.

Punctures that penetrate deep within the foot can involve structures such as joints, bones, and tendons. In these cases referral to a surgical facility may be warranted. Surgery may be the only option to gain access to these deeply infected structures. Surgery consists of removing dead tissue and establishing drainage. Even with surgery some infections deep in the foot cause permanent damage. Laminitis of the opposite limb can be a complication. Provide a support wrap to the opposite limb and follow guidelines as discussed in the laminitis section of this chapter. Most horses should receive a tetanus booster.

## Fracture of the Coffin Bone

Fractures of the coffin bone have been diagnosed in all horse breeds. These fractures can occur during exercise or by freak accident such as stepping on a rock or kicking an unforgiving surface. A common sign is acute lameness that may be non-weight bearing. There may be absolutely no swelling in the limb.

Definitive diagnosis is achieved by radio graphing the foot. Coffin bone fractures are further divided into several categories depending on the location of the fracture and joint involvement. Treatment is geared at immobilizing the hoof capsule by preventing hoof expansion. This can be accomplished in most cases with a bar shoe and clips. Surgery is another option for some horses.

Be aware that healing time can take up to a year. Most horses are put on strict stall confinement. Again, as with other debilitating foot problems, the opposite limb should be protected with support wraps and other methods to prevent laminitis. See the section of laminitis in this chapter for further information. Some horses suffer from chronic lameness, especially if the joint is involved.

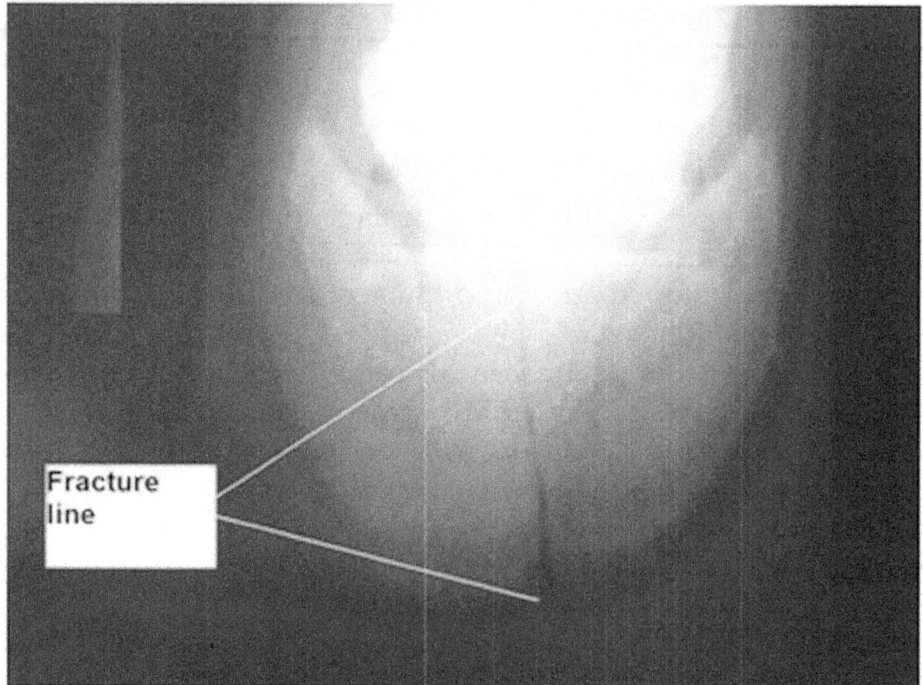

**Figure 8.14:** *Coffin Bone Fracture*

## Foot Abscess/Bruise

Hoof abscesses and bruises are typically not an emergency. Abscesses can have a slow progression to severe lameness. Lameness occurs due to the buildup of pus in the sensitive laminae of the foot. Bruises generally result in acute lameness that is not severe. Some bruises can turn into an abscess. In both cases the horse will generally allow the foot to be placed on the ground. Abscesses heal quicker if they are drained from the sole and bandaged appropriately.

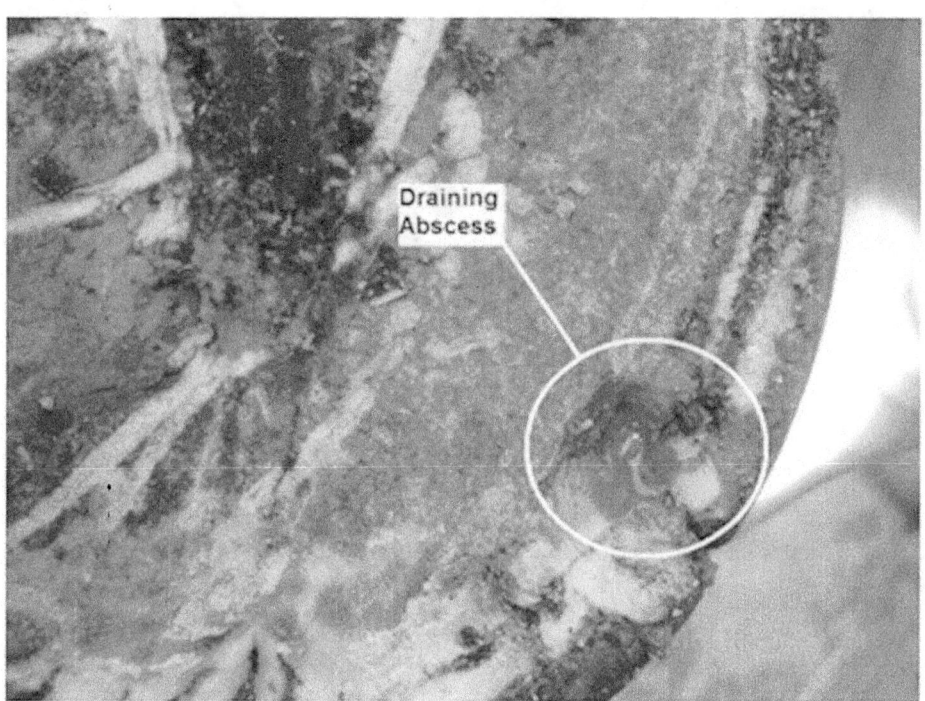

**Figure 8.15a:** *Abscess site*

Foot problems

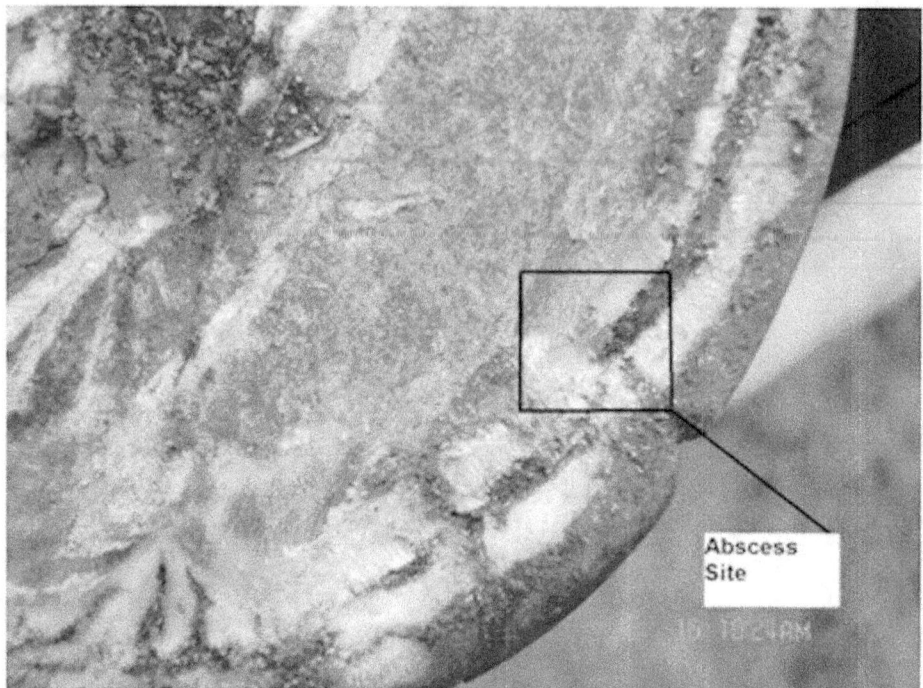

**Figure 8.15b:** *Abscess site opened*

We advise soaking the foot in warm water with Epsom salts. This can be done once daily as needed for several days. We save large IV fluid bags for soaking feet.

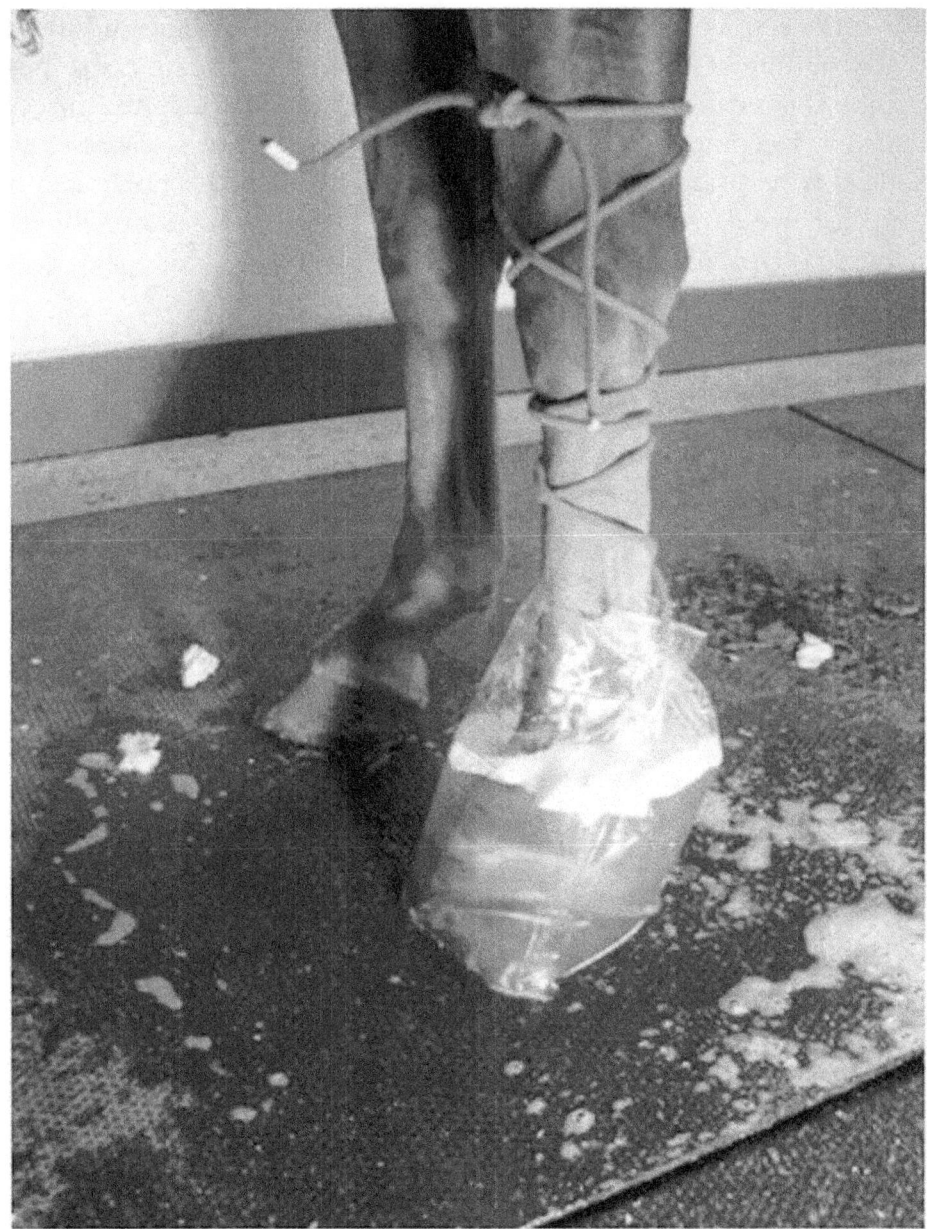

**Figure 8.16:** *Soaking foot in IV bag*

Hoof poultices are available for bandaging. Many farriers are capable of locating and draining abscesses. If the abscess is not drained from the solar surface, it will migrate along the path of least resistance up the hoof wall to rupture at the coronary band or heel bulb. Many horse people describe this as a *gravel*. Most horses recover rapidly once the abscess is drained. Keeping the opened abscessed area clean and dry with a bandage is necessary for prompt recovery. When the horse has been sound for five days off of pain medication, we recommend re-shoeing if the horse is typically shod.

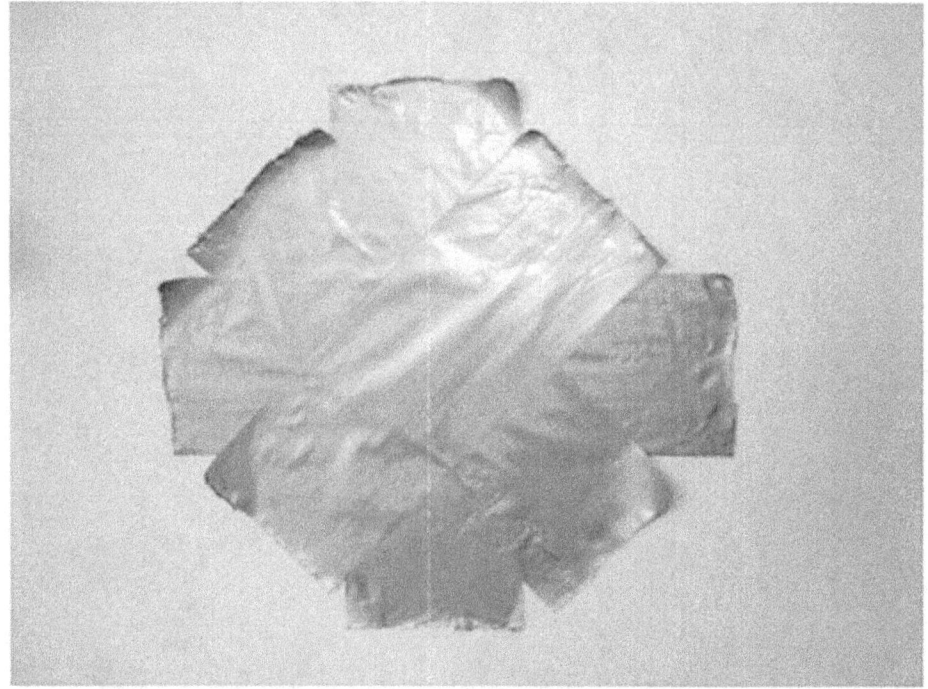

**Figure 8.17a:** *Preparing hoof bandage, two crosses of wide duct tape*

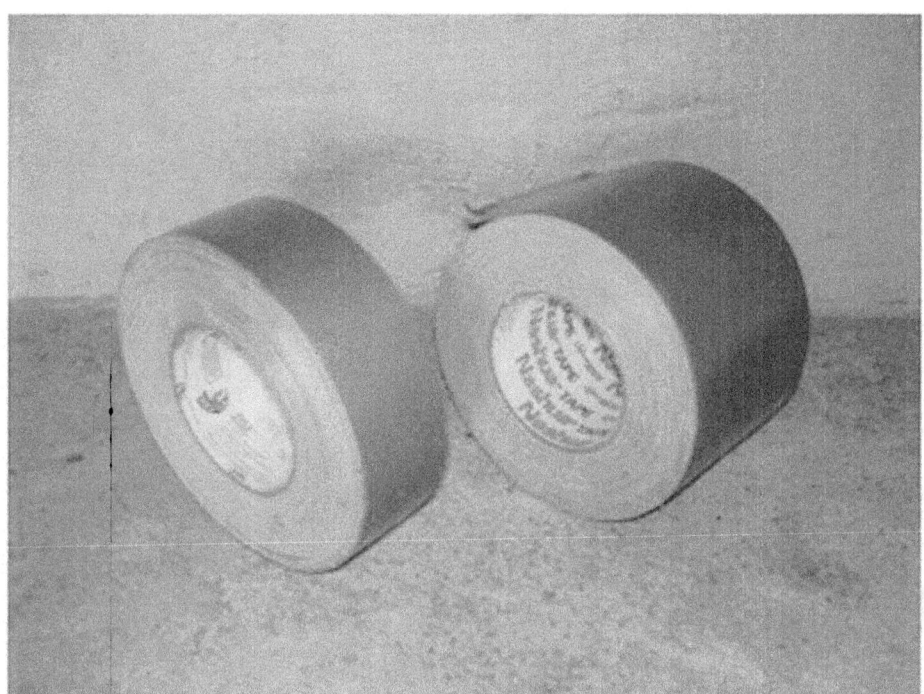

**Figure 8.17b:** *Wide versus normal duct tape*

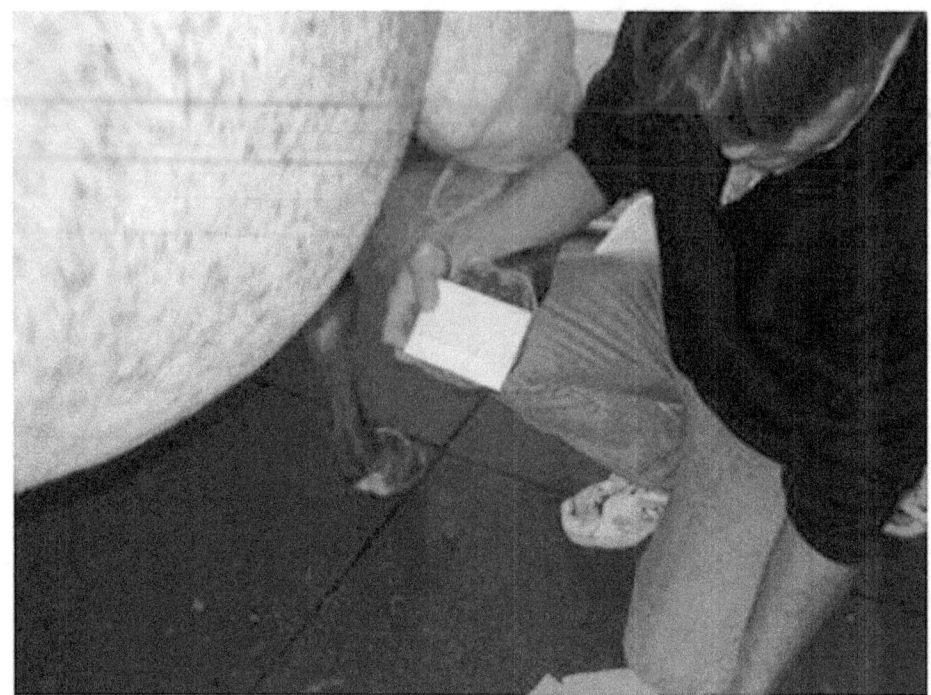

**Figure 8.17c:** *Apply dressing to hoof*

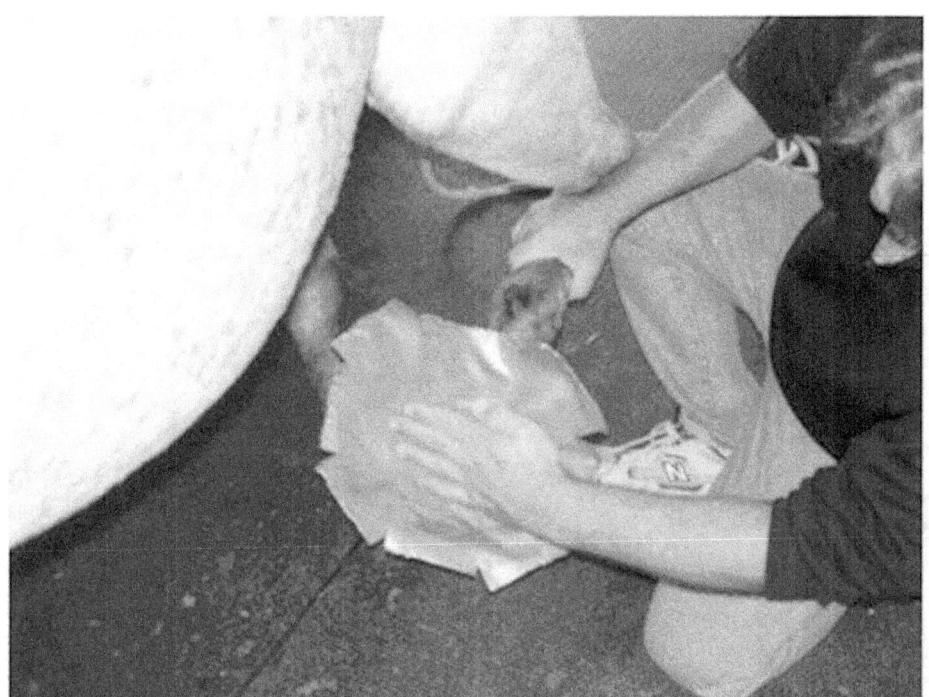

**Figure 8.17d:** *Apply duct tape crosses*

Foot problems

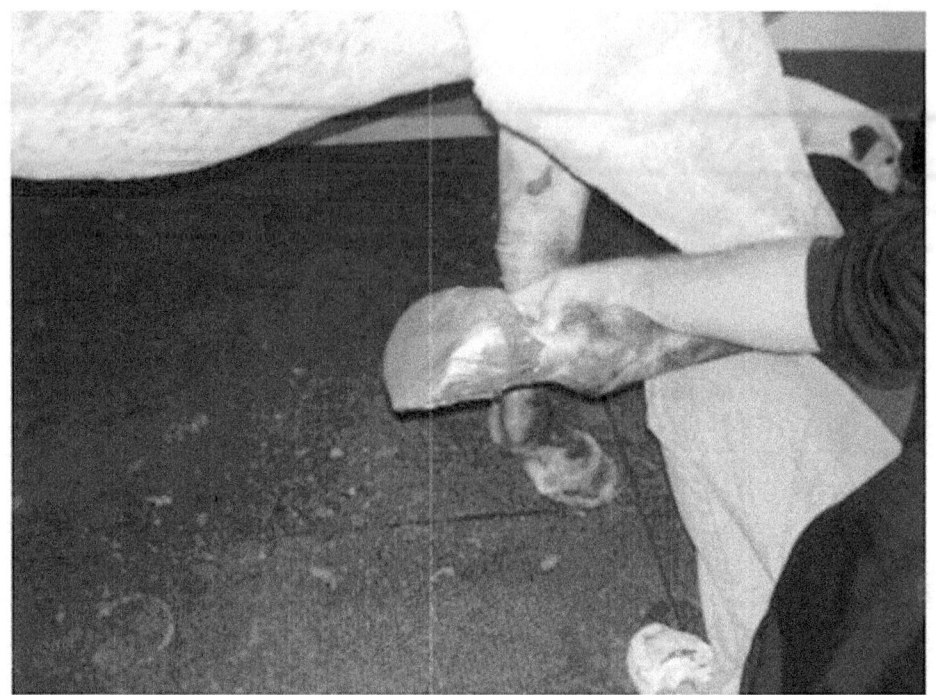

**Figure 8.17e:** *Fold edges up around hoof*

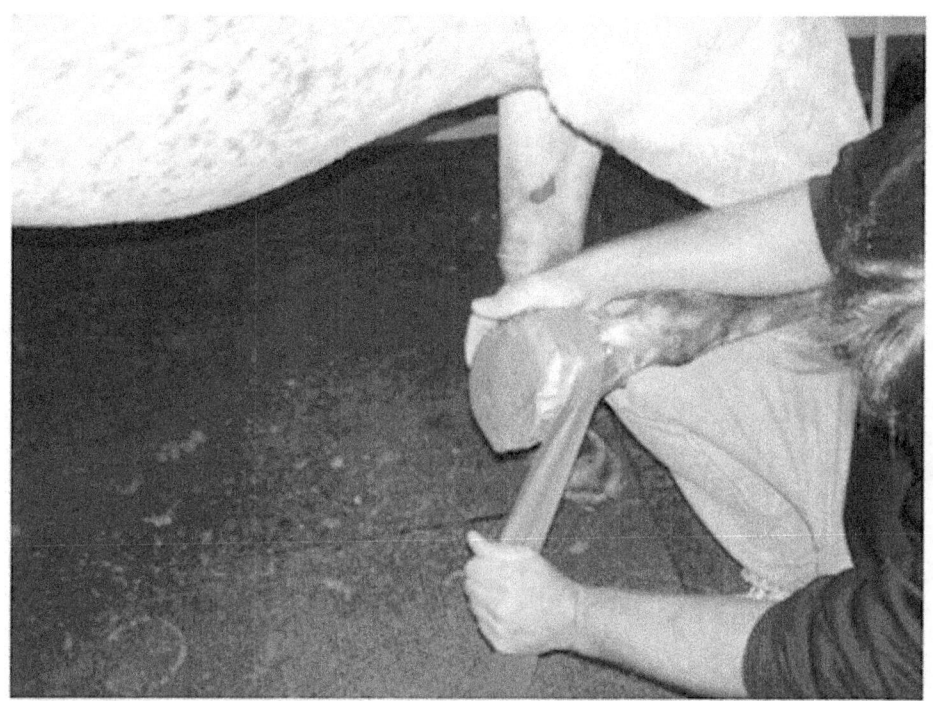

**Figure 8.17f:** *Secure bandage by wrapping snugly with narrow duct tape. Avoid pulling too tight at coronet*

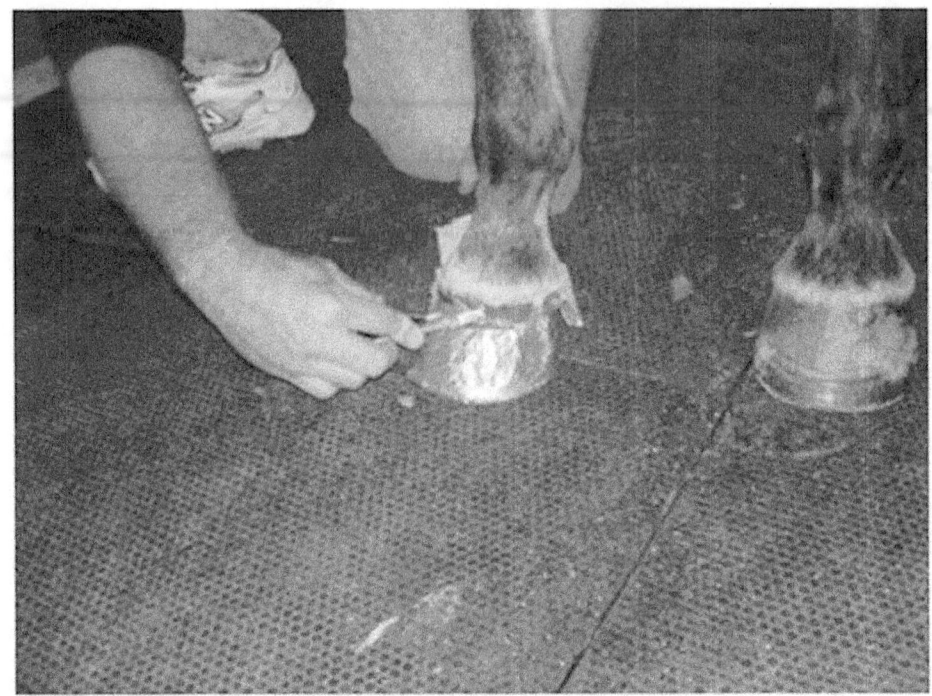

**Figure 8.17g:** *Remove excess tape with scissors, just below coronet*

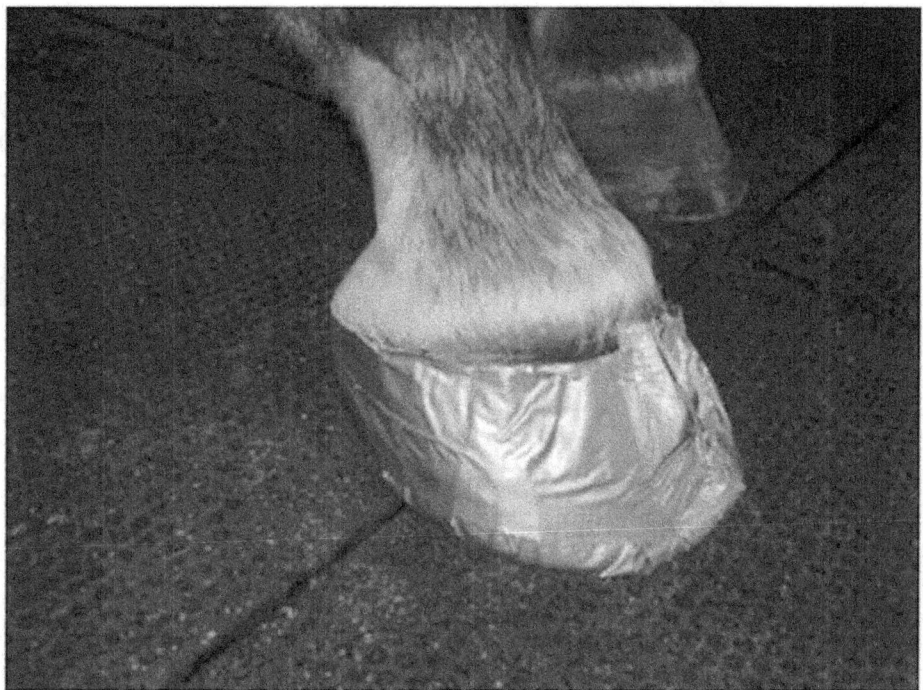

**Figure 8.17h:** *Finished bandage*

## Leg Fractures

Nowadays fractures are not necessarily an immediate death sentence. Techniques in surgery and stabilization have come a long way toward positive outcomes. Several variables play a role in the overall prognosis for leg fractures. That is to say not all fractures can be repaired and the same fractures in different horses can have very different outcomes. In this section we will cover what can be done immediately in the event of a fracture, and which fractures can have a favorable outcome.

Leg fractures cause horses to have non-weight bearing lameness if the fracture transverses the long axis of the bone. For instance, a chip off the corner of a long bone can be quite painful, but the horse will generally still bear weight into the limb. There may be obvious deformity of the limb and/or swelling at the fracture sight. Horses will not try to move or walk unless they are asked to do so.

If the fracture is high in the limb, there may not be discernable swelling, but contraction of the limb can occur. That is to say the limb may appear shorter than the opposite side. If you listen with a stethoscope, you may hear clicking or grinding when the leg is manipulated. If you determine that a fracture is likely to have occurred, call your veterinarian.

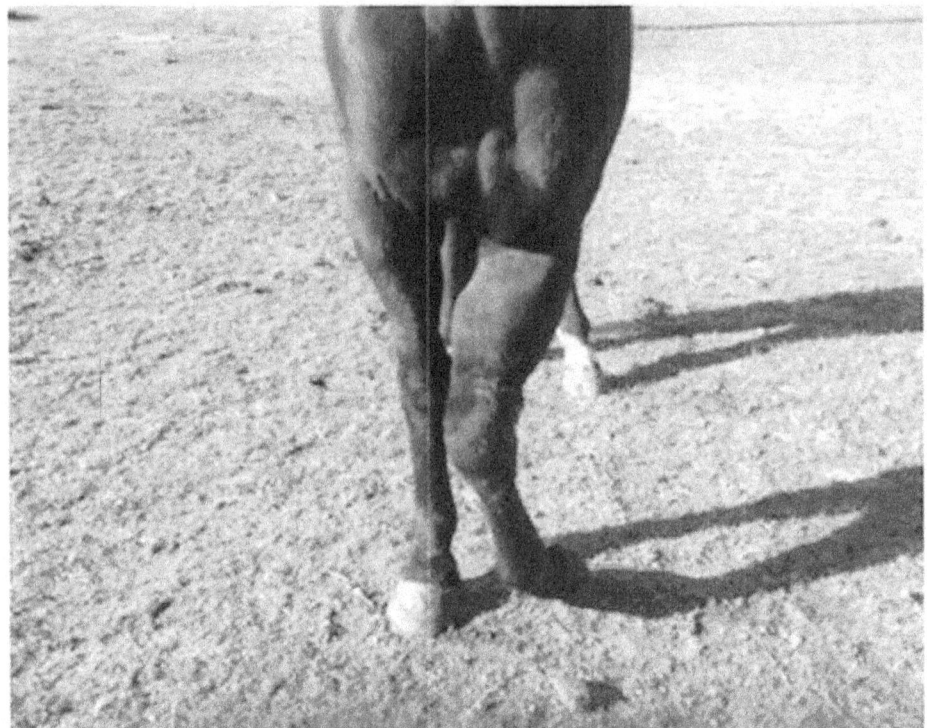

**Figure 8.18:** *Fractured Radius*

Immobilize the limb. Your veterinarian will decide which method is best to immobilize the limb. A *Robert Jones* bandage can be used for most any fracture. This is basically a full limb bandage that employs abundant soft padding the full length of the limb.

There are many types of splints and specialty braces that can be employed for various fractures. Handles from stall rakes or other similar tools can be incorporated into a padded leg wrap to provide stability.

Large diameter PVC pipe is also a common implement. All are geared at immobilization of the limb to prevent further damage and stabilize the limb to allow transport to a surgical facility. The jagged ends of a fractured bone can slice internal vessels like a knife if the limb is not stabilized.

As a general rule, fractures of bones closer to the body such as the femur, humerus, tibia, and radius have a poorer prognosis for repair and recovery than do fractures of the lower limb bones. Smaller, lightweight horses have a better prognosis for surgical repair of fractures. In any event, fractures are still a serious threat to your horse's life. Repair is often very costly and cannot be guaranteed. In many cases fracture repair is reserved for salvaging a breeding horse for future reproductive use. The risk of laminitis in the opposite limb is a concern during healing as well.

## Conclusion

This concludes the coverage of trauma emergencies. This chapter provided guidance on dealing with emergencies of the skin, hoof, and leg. These types of emergencies tend to be more visible and easier to diagnose than some of the emergencies that will be covered in the next chapter. The next chapter will cover emergencies of the eyes, nervous system, and metabolic system.

# Miscellaneous Emergencies

CHAPTER 9

This chapter will bring this book to a close with some of the emergencies that involve the eyes, the nervous system, and some metabolic emergencies such as poisonings, allergies, and muscle diseases. In some cases there is a clinical sign associated with an emergency that will key you in to the particular body system that is affected. In some cases the clinical signs can be vague as with muscle tremors or generalized weakness. At any rate, a complete physical exam is warranted and will often shed light on some of the more obscure disease states. The first section will cover emergencies of the eyes.

## Corneal Ulcers

A corneal ulcer is a relatively common condition among equines. Although in many cases they are readily treatable and have an excellent prognosis, there is no need to take a risk by waiting to have an eye problem examined. The anatomic position of the eye as well as its size on the side of the head can make it prone to injury. An ulcer can occur when the thin layer over the surface of the eye, also called the cornea, becomes scratched or abraded and subsequently develops an infection.

Clinically, these horses are experiencing pain in the eye area as evidenced by squinting and increased tear production. Upon closer examination one will see redness and/or swelling in the conjunctiva, which is the pink tissue under eyelids, and cloudiness of the cornea. Prompt treatment with topical antibiotics and possibly antifungal medication is necessary. Your veterinarian may perform a flouroscein dye stain of the eye. This dye helps to *light up* the ulcerated area or abraded area. Other stains can be performed to assess the eye's ability to fight off infection.

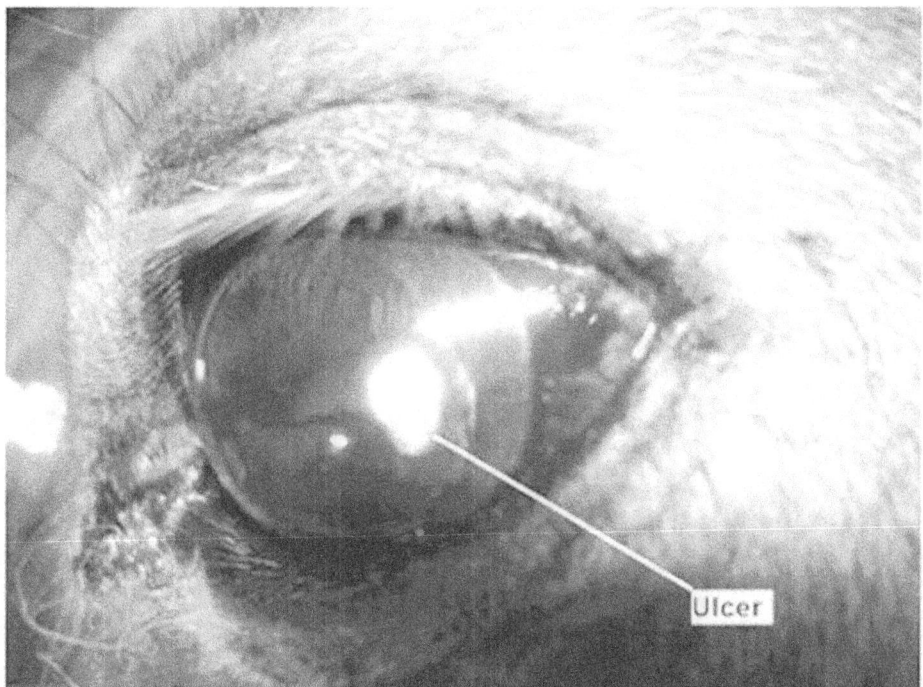

**Figure 9.1:** *Corneal Ulcer stained*

Location and size of the ulcer is noted early to gauge improvement or deterioration as treatment begins. Corneal ulcers can rapidly become infected with bacteria and or fungal organisms that can melt the cornea away. Since the average thickness of the cornea is only 1mm, this process can occur quite quickly and have devastating consequences. Horses that have melting ulcers usually will lose sight in the eye unless surgery is performed to treat the ulcer.

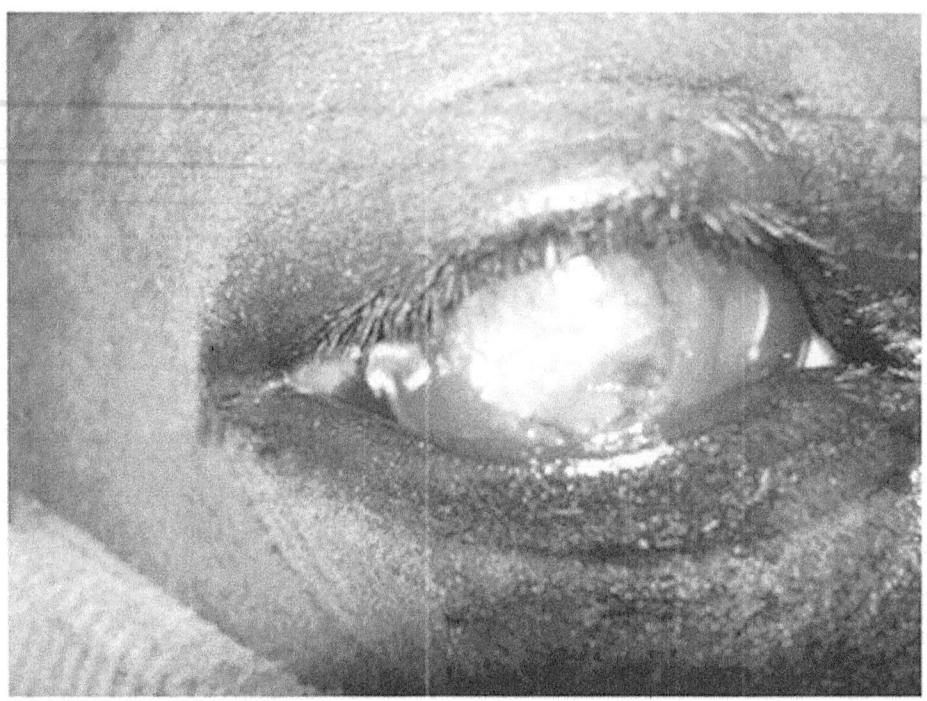

**Figure 9.2a:** *A conjunctival graft sewn to surface of cornea*

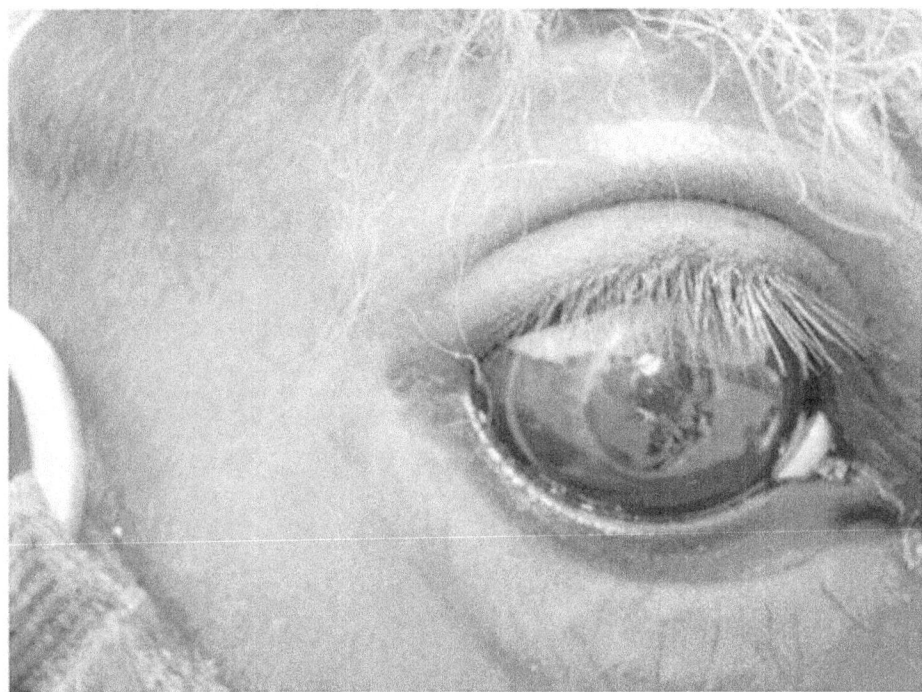

**Figure 9.2b:** *Same horse one year later*

Infection of the cornea is further complicated because the cornea does not have a good blood supply. Therefore, bacteria can grow and multiply within the corneal tissue without blood vessels bringing white blood cells to fight off the infection. In chronic ulcers, blood vessels actually grow from the outer areas of the eye over the cornea migrating to the affected area. This is known as neovascularization. In many cases, this new blood supply is still not sufficient so surgery is performed to bring a good blood supply as well as a protective covering to the ulcerated area.

Your veterinarian will decide on the antibiotic and frequency of application. Any eye ointment containing a corticosteroid such as dexamethasone should never be used on a corneal ulcer or other infection in the eye. For this reason, as with other medications, never use a left over eye ointment that was intended to treat another horse for a different condition.

Treating a horse's eye can be quite a challenge especially if the patient is fractious. For this reason, a device known as a sub-palpebral lavage system can be instilled in the eye by your veterinarian to facilitate treatment. This makes life easier for human and equine both!

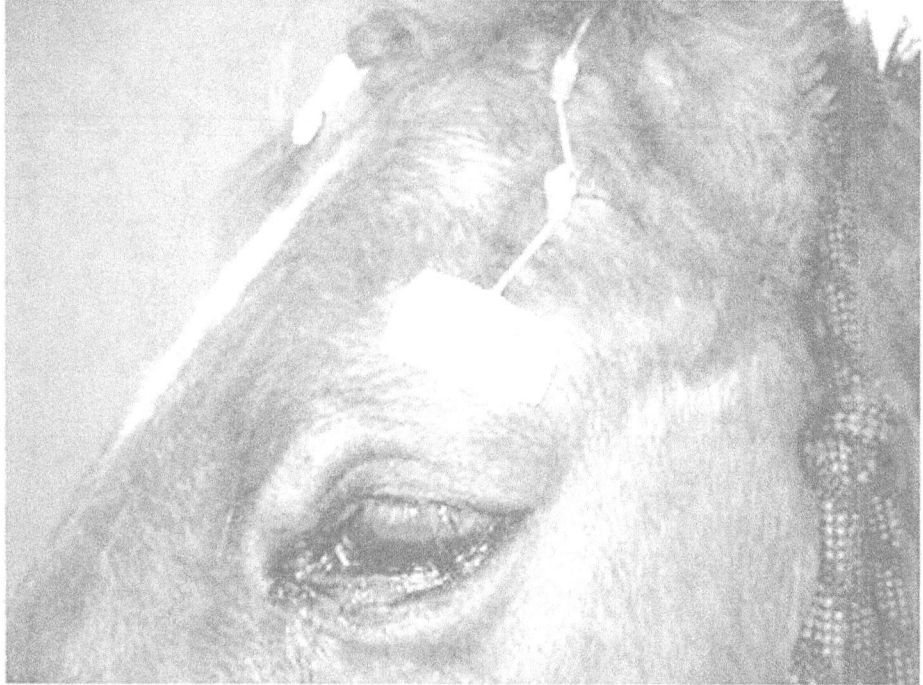

**Figure 9.3:** *A sub-palpebral lavage system to medicate the eye*

## Eyelid lacerations

Lacerations to the equine eyelid are common. The upper eyelid is routinely affected. Typically the horse jerks back quickly from a stimulus and catches the eyelid on an object such as a fence rail or handle to a bucket. In many cases, I will ask the client where the horse was when injured. Many times the owner will tell me that the horse was in a stall and that there was nothing that could injure them in the stall. I then probe and find that a bucket is hung in the stall by a metal handle. Upon close examination, a tinge of blood or even hairs can be seen on the handle. For this reason be careful if using buckets with handles.

Eyelid lacerations should be sutured as soon as possible, ideally within 12 hours. If left un-sutured, aside from being cosmetically unacceptable, the horse will now be prone to future eye problems. The hair from the flap may constantly rub the corneal surface thereby causing pain and possible infection. If there is a gap in the eyelid margin, there will be inadequate closing of the lid and spreading of tear film which will lead to dryness and keratitis in that particular area of the cornea. In the event that your horse experiences an eyelid laceration, apply triple antibiotic ointment to the area and alert your veterinarian.

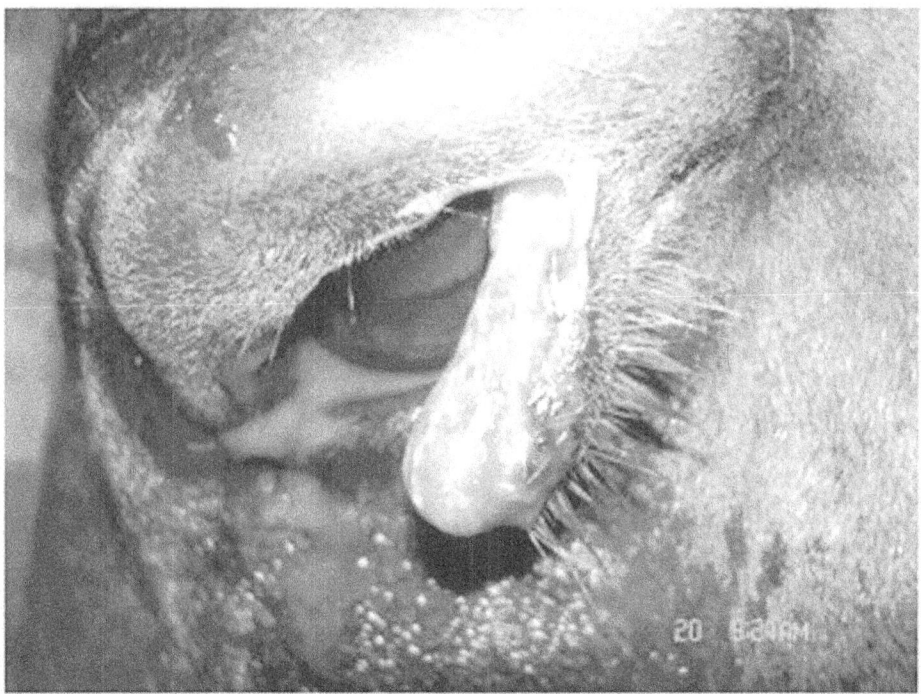

**Figure 9.4a:** *Common type of Eyelid laceration*

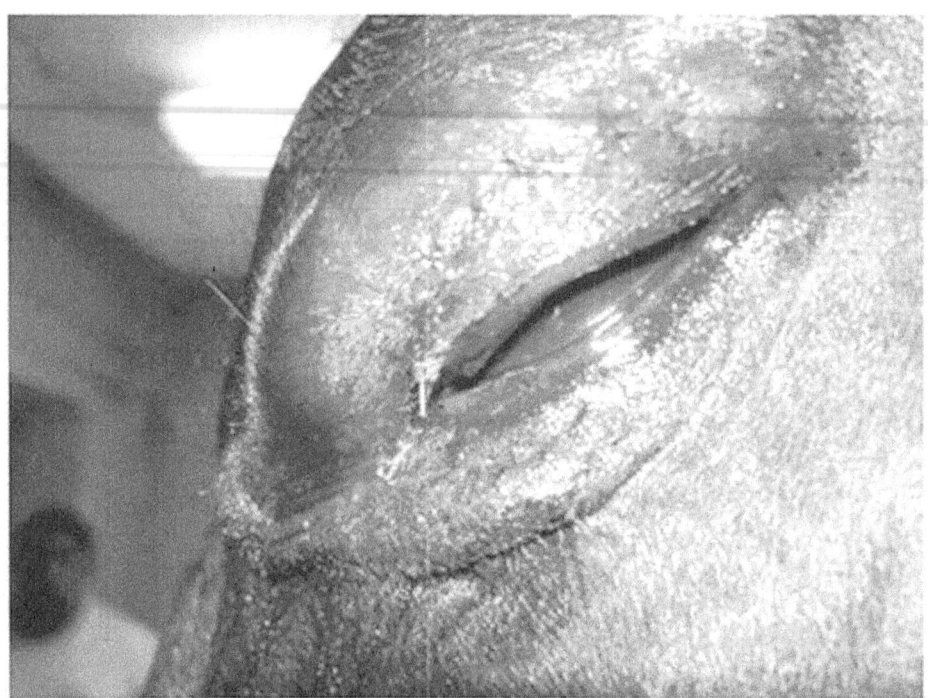

**Figure 9.4b:** *Eyelid immediately after suturing*

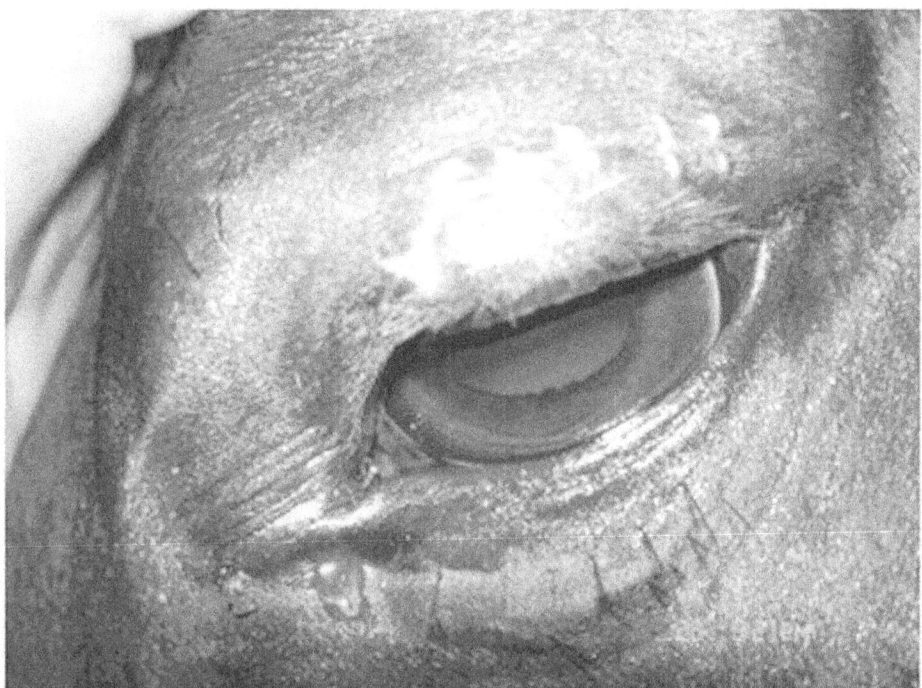

**Figure 9.4c:** *Eyelid laceration at suture removal*

## Equine Recurrent Uveitis

Equine Recurrent Uveitis (ERU) is a common eye disease in horses. It is also referred to as Moon Blindness. It is recurrent in nature, meaning the horse will be affected on numerous different occasions. Most times an episode can be predicated by a stressful event such as de-worming, vaccination, or travel.

The uveal tract is a network of tissue and blood vessels within and behind the iris inside the eye. When this area becomes inflamed, the normal barrier to keep blood borne products out of the eye is breached thereby letting blood, bacteria, and other circulatory antigens into the eye. This in turn sets up an immune response which further exacerbates the inflammation within the eye.

Early signs of uveitis include dilation and redness of the internal vessels. This can progress to squinting and excess tears flowing from the eye(s). The anterior chamber of the eye may become cloudy from the debris leaking from the blood. The surface of the cornea may become cloudy and blue in appearance. These are the clinical signs to be aware of with uveitis. It should be noted that uveitis can occur due to other eye diseases, such as ulcers or injury. Uveitis in these cases appears to occur as single entities and do not recur. ERU episodes can lead to irreversible damage with in the eyes and subsequently end up in blindness.

Treatment of ERU is geared at controlling pain and reducing inflammation within the eye. Careful staining of the eye with flouroscein stain is important to rule out any corneal ulceration and infection. As long as no ulceration or infection is present, corticosteroids can be used in the eye to reduce pain and inflammation. Systemic steroids can be used as well but are less effective. Surgical implantation of cyclosporine in the eye has shown promising results for many horses. Over time with repeated episodes, some horses develop irreversible damage to the eye which requires removal of the eye to alleviate pain and infection.

If you suspect your horse to be suffering from uveitis contact your vet and discuss your findings. Be sure to give a history of any stressful events that could have triggered an episode. Protect your horse's eyes from insects and sunlight with a fly mask. It is not wise to administer any previously prescribed ophthalmic ointments before the eye can be stained.

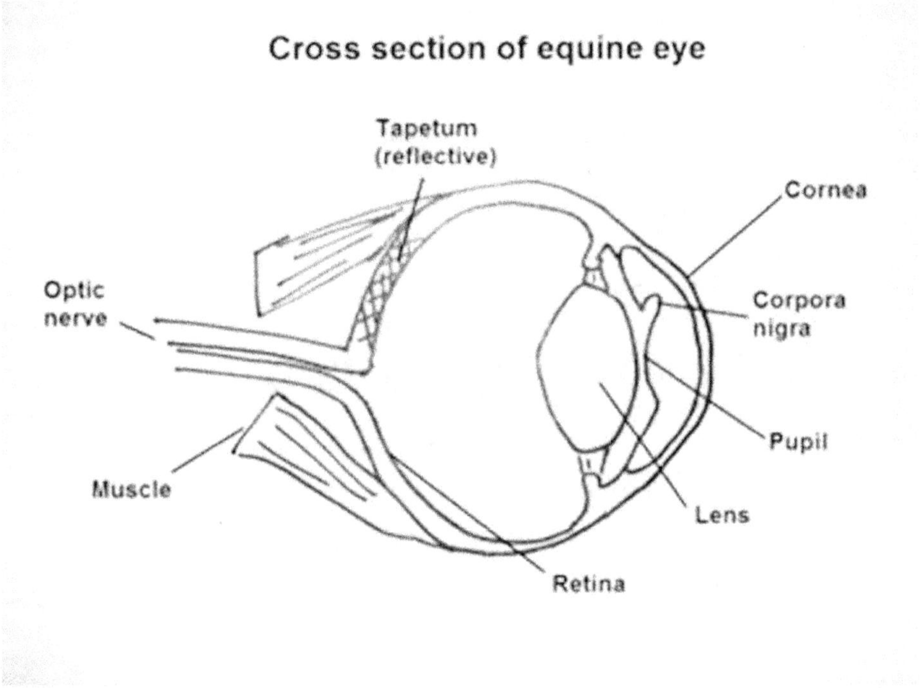

**Cross section of equine eye**

**Figure 9.5:** *Equine eye anatomy*

# Seizures

Seizures can occur in horses at any age. A seizure happens when the electrical activity in the brain is compromised. In some cases there may be local muscle twitching in one area of the body. In other cases, the horse may go down. In these cases, the horse is unresponsive to all external stimuli. Unless trained to treat a seizing horse, it is probably best to keep your distance as the flailing horse may injure you. The horse may also injure itself so only intervene if absolutely necessary to prevent the horse for severe injury. At no time should you place yourself at risk.

Seizures can occur from swellings in the brain caused by infections or tumors. Seizures may also result from electrolyte imbalances such as low blood sodium and blood sugars. Several diagnostic tests are available including blood sampling, head radiographs (x-rays), neurological tests,

CT scans, and spinal taps. If an entity causing the seizure can be isolated, treatment may be possible.

Sedative-type drugs can be used to stop a seizure in progress. Some drugs can be used to help control future seizures, but are unreliable at best. Remember to keep track of seizure episodes by recording when they occur and if they are related to a particular stimulus. Determining the exact cause for seizures can be quite difficult and expensive.

## Exertional Rhabdomyolysis (Tying up)

This disease is known also as Monday morning disease, azoturia, setfast, and tying up. Affected horses will typically show signs after exercise. These signs include:

- Hard, cramped muscles
- Muscle stiffness and pain especially in the hind limbs
- Profuse sweating
- High heart and respiratory rates
- Very reluctant to walk or move
- Clinical signs of colic may also be present

If your horse appears to be tying up, allow the horse to rest and do not try to force walking. Often times your vet can administer potent pain relief such as flunixin meglumine, xylazine, or detomidine. In some cases, on oral dose of fluid therapy and electrolytes is needed via nasogastric tube. Your veterinarian may also elect to draw a blood sample to assess the circulating enzymes in the bloodstream. These are good indicators for the extent of muscle damage. In some cases your horse may need fluid therapy to correct dehydration and protect the kidneys from damage due to high levels of circulating muscle protein (myosin) in the blood.

Horses that experience exertional rhabdomyolysis are usually unfit for the exercise they had performed prior to the episode. Therefore, to prevent further attacks a slowly increasing exercise regimen should be implemented. A change in diet is also beneficial. Horses prone to exertional rhabdomyolysis should be fed a high-fiber, high-fat, low-starch diet. These diets can be commercially prepared to meet your horse's exact requirements. We also recommend that horses be fed electrolyte supplements in their feed or water before a scheduled event.

## Polysaccharide Storage Myopathy

This disease is primarily seen in Quarter horse breeds. It can also be seen in draft and warmblood breeds. It is similar in appearance to exertional rhabdomyolysis. The clinical signs can vary from pain and stiffness to reluctance to move. Some horses also appear weak and will collapse with out being able to get back up. Generally 5-10 year old horses are first to show signs. There also appears to be a genetic link. There is currently not a genetic test for the disease. Testing now involves obtaining a muscle biopsy from the horse and using special stains to see the abnormal changes in the muscle cells.

If affected, keep the horse turned out. If the horse is down, try using a tarp or similar sheeting to keep the eyes from injury. The affected horses should be fed a low sugar, low starch diet that has added fat for energy. The diet should also be high in fiber. Nowadays horse feeds have become quite specialized, so investigate a commercial preparation that may be available.

## Hyperkalemic Periodic Paralysis

Hyperkalemic Periodic Paralysis (HYPP) is a genetic disease. Most anyone that has been in the horse industry for a while will have heard of this disease. The disease was first discovered in the 1980s affecting Quarter horses that shared a common ancestor -- the famous sire Impressive. Due to Impressive's favorable attributes of having muscular offspring, he was extremely sought after as a breeding stallion. Unfortunately, he passed on a genetic mutation that causes the disease.

Not all of the descendants are affected in the same way. Some horses carry a homozygous gene (2 copies) whereas others may be heterozygous (1 copy) and still others may not have any copy of the gene. Genetic testing has been developed to definitively determine which horses carry the genes. Those horses are then listed with the AQHA on their registration as carriers. It is possible to eliminate the disease by not breeding carriers but this has actually not occurred. In fact, over the years, an increasing number of horses have been shown to carry the gene. One statistic shows that approximately 160,000 horses are known to carry the gene. This has likely occurred since the breeders still want the desirable well muscled horse. The AQHA has now stated that having a horse that carries the HYPP gene to be undesirable.

The clinical signs of HYPP can range from mild twitching to full paralysis. Some horses may exhibit abnormal breathing and/or respiratory noise due to paralysis in the larynx. Horses may tremble, sweat, and experience uncontrollable twitching. One client described to me that when his horse was having an attack it looked like mice were crawling under his horse's skin all over his body. In extreme cases, the horse can die.

Treatment is aimed at prevention by administering daily medication (acetazolamide) to help clear the body of excess calcium. In the event the horse is suffering from an episode, you may administer additional acetazolamide as prescribed by your veterinarian along with a sugar such as corn syrup to help the muscle cell stabilize. Light exercise can also benefit the horse if an attack is eminent. In severe episodes, obviously call your veterinarian who can administer intravenous treatments to stabilize the muscle cells. As with some other metabolic diseases, a special diet that is low in potassium is recommended for these horses.

If your horse is confirmed to be positive for HYPP, alert your vet before any procedure that would require sedation or anesthesia. These events could stimulate an attack. Keep your horse protected from injury during an attack. In particular protect the head and eyes. Do not allow the horse to lie on one side for extended periods of time. Pull the front leg that is next to the ground as far forward as possible to protect against pressure damage to the nerves. If the horse is flailing, do not attempt any of these procedures until the horse can relax. Remember that you will not be able to help your horse if you get knocked out!

## Poisonous plants and Toxins

There is a long list of plants that can be poisonous to horses. Some of these plants cause mild to moderate illness whereas others can be fatal. Your horse may experience different exposure to different plants depending on the geography and climate of your area. We recommend that you contact your extension agency to determine what plants are deemed hazardous in your area and identify and remove them. There are also complete manuals available that describe how to identify poisonous plants and the symptoms that may occur.

In general, horses do not usually tend to ingest poisonous plants because they are mostly bitter and unpalatable. Horses that are stalled or fed mainly hay may be more at risk if turned out to pasture because they may sample several types of plants. If the pasture is not maintained, it can become overwhelmed with poor grazing plants and poisonous weeds may be ingested.

When a poisoning is suspected, early treatment is important to reduce the amount of toxin(s) absorbed into the body. Activated charcoal and mineral oil is typically administered via nasogastric tube to help absorb toxins from the stomach contents and intestines. Mineral oil acts as a cathartic to help speed up the transit of digestive contents through the gut. If the toxic principle is known, an antidote or pharmaceutical drug is sometimes available to reverse the negative effects of the toxin. If the toxin is being absorbed through the skin, prompt washing with a dish detergent with copious rinsing is advised.

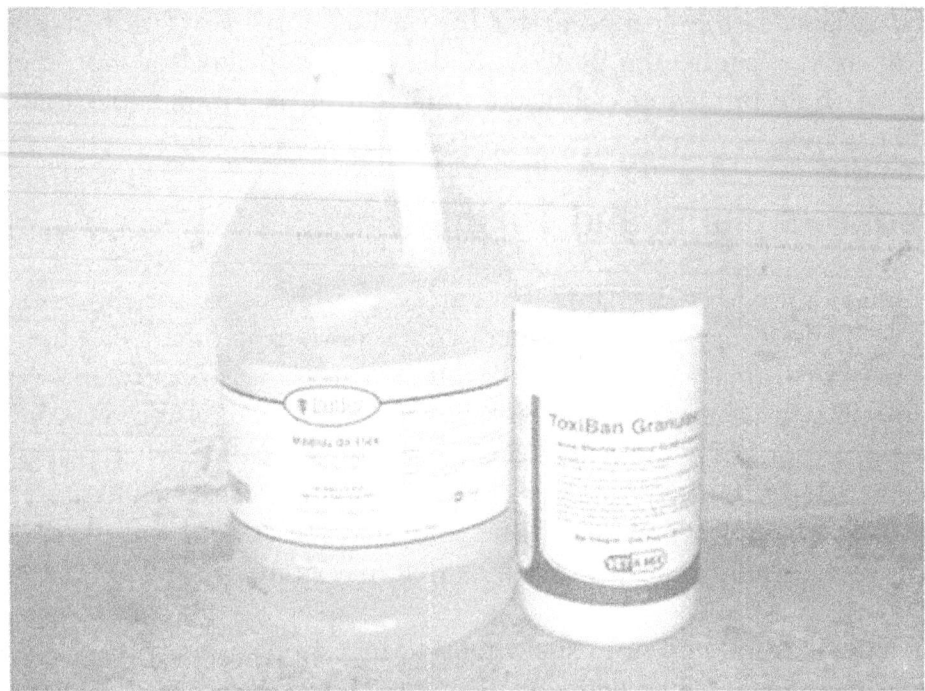

**Figure 9.6:** *Activated charcoal and mineral oil*

## Heat stress/ Anhidrosis

Heat stress or heat stroke can occur in any age horse particularly during exercise in hot/humid weather. Horses confined to small, unventilated areas such as a stall or trailer during hot weather are more at risk. Horses that are not in good physical shape as well as overweight and heavily muscled horses that cannot dissipate heat rapidly are at a higher risk. Flared nostrils with rapid breathing as well as reluctance to move and generalized weakness are predominant physical signs. Body temperature may soar as high as 110F. Internal organ damage can occur rapidly so prompt treatment is necessary to prevent secondary problems.

Firstly, cool the horse as quick as possible with running water from a hose. Cooling will occur quicker if the water is run continuously for 20 –30 minutes. In addition to water, isopropyl alcohol can be poured over the neck and back to enhance cooling by evaporation. Higher humidity slows evaporation from sweating so run fans on the horse to help evaporative processes that will additionally cool the horse. Avoid draping the horse with wet towels or sheets, as this will trap body heat. Instead use a sweat scraper, and allow the horse to dry. The evaporative process will release heat from the horse quicker.

Your veterinarian may elect to provide intravenous fluids to aid in electrolyte and fluid replacement. Administration of flunixin meglumine is helpful to reduce fever and treat any endotoxemia.

Anhidrosis is the inability to sweat. This can develop over time especially in horses that are exposed to high heat and humidity for a long period of time. There is a diagnostic test to determine if the horse is anhidrotic. The test consists of an injection of epinephrine in the dermis of the skin. Normal horses will sweat at the injection site within 30 minutes. Anhidrotic horses have signs similar to heat exhaustion as described above. Heavy panting and increased exercise intolerance are noted.

Management of the condition is required. Obviously avoid riding during the hottest weather and high humidity. Use fans with misters to keep the horses cool. Dietary modifications that reduce overall concentrate in the diet have shown to be helpful. Supplementation or access to salt and electrolytes is important as well. Drug therapy for anhidrosis has not yet been approved with controlled studies. Discuss these treatments with your veterinarian.

## Allergic reactions

An allergic reaction occurs when the horse is exposed to an allergen that causes a heightened immune response. These allergens can be inhaled, injected, eaten and in some cases caused by something coming in contact with the skin. Some horses, like people, are more prone to allergies than others. Fortunately, most allergic reactions are mild and pass without much concern or need for treatment. In rare cases, an anaphylactic reaction could occur that can result in death if not treated immediately.

Obstruction of the airway and circulatory collapse can lead to death if not reversed immediately. The treatment of choice is epinephrine. Refer to the respiratory chapter for guidelines to handle anaphylactic reactions.

Raised nodules in the skin that can cover only part or the whole body characterize hives and other skin conditions and may be the result of an allergic reaction. These conditions are covered in chapter 8.

## Sudden Death

The sudden or unexpected death in the horse occurs from time to time. Sometimes the horse may be found in the pasture or in the stall with no apparent cause of death. A necropsy exam can be performed in some cases to detect the actual cause of death. Sudden death occurring during exercise is most often attributed to internal bleeding or conditions of heart failure. Sudden death that occurs any other time can be due to a variety of conditions. Sometimes there may be an acute colic episode that involves torsion of the root of the mesentery. Electrocution and lightening strike can also be causes of sudden death.

Inspect the surroundings for clues such as what the horse had been eating during the time before death. Are there any external wounds or punctures? Was there any sign of struggle? Even with a thorough necropsy examination, the cause of death can remain a mystery. Consult with your veterinarian for the best course of action. If other horses are on the premises, you may be inclined to have a necropsy performed by a qualified veterinary pathologist to determine if the cause of death could be prevented. Contact your insurance company immediately before the horse is buried, in case any samples or a necropsy is required.

## Conclusion

While the scope of this book has been geared toward the treatment of horses during emergencies, the thought process of preventing emergencies has been addressed as much as possible. This book was written to help the horse owner recognize what an emergency is, how to prepare the animal for treatment, and what to expect during and after treatment for the specific problem. This book is not a replacement for quality veterinary care when an emergency arises. Only a licensed veterinarian is legally capable of prescribing and treating an ailing horse.

Become familiar with the different types of emergencies that may occur so that, if possible, they can be prevented altogether. If an emergency arises, do not delay treatment. The sooner any emergency is addressed, the better the outcome.

# Index

2nd degree heart block ............................. 5
abdominocentesis ............................. 125, 133
Abortion ............................................... 69
abscesses ......... 28, 29, 32, 155, 185, 206, 209
activated charcoal ................................ 135
afterbirth ........................................... 33, 70
Anaphylaxis ..................................... 46, 145
Anhidrosis ...................................... 234, 235
Anthelmintics .................................... 52, 57
antibiotics ........ 32, 47, 70, 100, 140, 148, 155, 156, 157, 205, 220
anticonvulsant .................................... 100
Ascarids ............................................. 55
asphyxiation ....................................... 135
aspiration pneumonia ..................... 127, 154
azoturia ............................................. 230
Bacitracin ........................................... 30
Banamine ....................................... 31, 126
barking foal ......................................... 99
barrel ................................................. 16
bismuth ............................................. 135
blood loss ........................................... 163
blood pressure .................................. 6, 100
Bot fly ................................................ 56
Botulism ............................................. 45
bronchospasms .................................... 153
Burns ........................................... 157, 178
bute ................................... See Phenylbutazone
camped in ............................................ 15
cannula .............................................. 125
capillary refill time ............................. 6, 68
carpus .......................................... 104, 106
cellulitis ............................................. 179
chest..4, 16, 94, 138, 146, 150, 153, 154, 155, 156, 166, 180
Choke ......................................... 135, 146
Chronic Obstructive Pulmonary Disease 151
circulation ...................................... 6, 133
Coastal Bermuda hay ........................... 130
coffin bone ............................ 188, 192, 205
Coggins Test .................................... 41, 60
Colic ..................... 98, 101, 115, 119, 191
colostrum ........... 33, 64, 91, 99, 101, 112, 113
COPD ............................................... 151

corneal ulcer .................................. 220, 223
Corpora Nigra ....................................... 12
deformities ........................... 98, 103, 106, 164
de-wormer ............................. 55, 57, 58, 59
deworming ....................................... 52, 55
dexamethasone ............................... 192, 223
diarrhea ............ 45, 55, 98, 100, 101, 102, 140
digestive tract ........................... 9, 21, 55, 129
digital pulses ............................. 19, 190, 191
digital thermometer ................................. 2
dummy foal .......................................... 99
Dystocia ............................................... 70
Eastern Equine Encephalitis ............... 41, 64
EEE ....................................... 41, 42, 64
EHV1 ................................................. 43
EHV4 ................................................. 43
EIA .................................................... 60
Elastikon ............................................. 29
electrolytes ...................... 140, 156, 230, 235
endophyte fescue hay ............................. 64
endotoxemia ................................. 191, 235
endotoxic shock .................................. 134
enteritis ............................................. 102
entrapment ................................... 128, 133
epinephrine .................... 46, 145, 235, 236
Epistaxis ........................................... 149
EPM ............................................. 46, 53
Equine Herpes Virus - Type 1 ................. 43
Equine Herpes Virus – Type 1 ................. 64
Equine Infectious Anemia ...................... 60
Equine Influenza .................................. 42
Equine Protozoal Myelitis ...................... 46
Equine Recurrent Uveitis ...................... 227
Equine Rhinopneumonitis ...................... 70
Equine Viral Arteritis ............................ 45
Eqvalan .............................................. 59
ERU ........................................... 227, 228
Ethmoid hematomas ............................ 149
Exertional Rhabdomyolysis ................... 230
extensor tendons ................................. 163
fecal material ....................................... 21
Fenbendazole ....................................... 58
fetus .............................................. 69, 70
first aid kit .................................... 27, 160

flank .................................................. 3, 9, 16, 126
flatworm ...................................................... 54
flexor tendon ..................................... 163, 164
Flunixin.............................................. 126, 147
founder ................................................. 83, 134
fractures ...................................... 205, 217, 218, 219
Furacin ointment.......................................... 30
gestation ..................................... 63, 64, 70, 98
gum color ......................................... 6, 122, 157
guttural pouch ......................................... 150
heat stroke ............................................... 234
Heaves ........................................................ 151
Hematomas.................................................. 180
hernia ............................................. 67, 111, 133
Hives .......................................................... 178
hoof punctures ........................................... 203
hydrogen peroxide ................................. 30, 161
Hyperkalemic Periodic Paralysis ...... 146, 231
Hypoxic Ischemic Encephalopathy .......... 99
HYPP........................................ 146, 231, 232
IgG test................................................... 91, 94
Impaction ................................................... 129
impaction colic ........................................... 130
infection..14, 30, 48, 49, 65, 69, 70, 102, 112, 131, 147, 150, 153, 160, 164, 166, 177, 178, 179, 180, 181, 192, 205, 220, 223, 225, 228
intramuscular injections ............................ 47
Ivermectin .................................................... 59
jaundice ...................................................... 113
keratitis ...................................................... 225
laceration ................... 159, 160, 163, 177, 225
laminitis ....134, 135, 164, 189, 190, 191, 192, 203, 205, 206, 219
Laryngeal Paralysis .................................... 145
**Lax flexor tendons** ................................. 103
lower respiratory disease........................... 150
lung fields ............................................. 3, 155
lung worms .................................................. 57
lymph node .......................................... 14, 147
Mare Rejection ..................................... 98, 112
meconium ....................................... 33, 94, 101
Monday morning disease .......................... 230
Moon Blindness ......................................... 227
Moxidectin ................................................... 59
mucous membranes...6, 9, 68, 102, 113, 126, 133, 140, 178

nasogastric feeding tube........................... 100
nasogastric tube126, 127, 130, 131, 133, 134, 135, 139, 230, 233
nasolacrimal duct ....................................... 13
navel ............................... 34, 39, 79, 88, 93, 111
navel ill....................................................... 112
necropsy ............................................. 113, 236
Neomycin ..................................................... 30
Neonatal Isoerythrolysis ........................... 113
Neonatal Maladjustment Syndrome......98, 99
neovascularization ..................................... 223
NI 113
NMS..................................................... 99, 100
Nolvasan ....................................... 30, 34, 161
oribatid mite ............................................... 54
oxytetracycline ................................... 104, 106
packed cell volume ................................... 123
Panacur ....................................................... 58
Panancur ..................................................... 55
Paraphimosis ............................................... 65
parasites ..................... 21, 53, 54, 57, 59, 60
parasitology ................................................. 53
patent urachus .......................................... 111
Penile Hematoma ....................................... 67
Peripartum Asphyxia.................................. 99
Phenylbutazone .................................... 30, 147
pinworms .................................................... 57
placenta.70, 71, 79, 81, 83, 85, 86, 92, 93, 99, 113
Placenta Previa ........................................... 79
Placentitis ................................................... 70
pleuritis ............................................. 153, 154
pleuropneumonia ...................................... 153
Pneumabort-K™ ......................................... 43
Pneumobort-K ............................................ 64
pneumonia .99, 102, 140, 142, 147, 151, 153, 156, 157
Pneumothorax................................... 155, 156
poisonous plants ................................. 36, 233
Polymyxin ................................................... 30
Polysaccharide Storage Myopathy............ 231
Potomac Horse Fever ................... 45, 53, 191
Praziquantel ................................................ 59
premature ................... 63, 69, 70, 98, 99, 101
proud flesh .......................................... 30, 180
pulmonary edema ..................................... 157
Pulmonary Hemmorhage ......................... 150

purpura hemorrhagica .................................. 147
Pyrantal pamoate/tartrate ............................ 58
quarantine ............................................ 41, 44, 61
Quest ............................................................. 59
Rabies ..................................................... 44, 64
RAO ........................................... 151, 152, 153
Rectal Bleeding ........................................... 68
rectal exam ................................................ 122
Recurrent Airway Obstruction ................ 151
Redbag ........................................................ 79
regurgitation ............................................. 127
respiration rate ................. 102, 122, 133, 191
respiratory rate ......................... 3, 100, 126
rhinopneumonitis ...................................... 43
Rhodococcus ............................................ 155
Robert Jones bandage .............................. 218
roundworms .............................................. 55
rump ............................................................ 16
Safegard ....................................................... 58
Salmonella ................................................ 102
sand colic ........................................... 131, 132
Scrotal hernia ............................................. 67
SDF ............................................................ 156
Seizures .................................................... 229
Sepsis ................................................... 98, 101
septic shock ................................................ 68
setfast ........................................................ 230
Shipping fever ......................................... 147
shock ................ 127, 133, 150, 157, 163, 178
silver nitrate ............................................. 112
skin tent .................................... 8, 122, 126, 140
skin worms ................................................. 57
smoke inhalation ..................................... 157
Snake Bite ................................................ 148
SPAOD ....................................... 151, 152, 153
standing exam ........................................... 15
stethoscope 3, 4, 10, 122, 140, 146, 150, 153, 154, 155, 156, 218
stomach ulceration ........................... 32, 141
stomach worms .......................................... 57

Strangles .......................................... 43, 145, 147
strangulated bowel .................................... 133
strangulating colic ............................. 133, 191
Streptococcus ................................... 43, 147
Strongid .................................................. 58, 60
strongyles ............................................... 56, 59
submandibular area .................................... 14
sub-palpebral lavage system ...................... 224
Sudden death ............................................ 236
Summer Pasture Associated Obstructive Pulmonary Disease ............................... 151
Synchronous diaphragmatic flutter .......... 156
tapeworm ................................................ 54, 59
Tetanus .................................................... 44, 64
threadworm ................................................. 57
Thumps .................................................... 156
Tooth Abscess .......................................... 150
torsion ............................... 87, 128, 133, 236
tracheal collapse ....................................... 146
tracheotomy .............. 142, 144, 145, 146, 148
twinning ..................................................... 63
twitch ........................................... 27, 65, 112
twitching .................................................... 27
Tying up .................................................... 230
umbilicus ............................... 79, 111, 112
upper respiratory disease .................... 14, 142
urachus ..................................................... 111
urticaria .................................................... 178
vaccination ........ 41, 42, 44, 45, 52, 60, 61, 227
Vaginal Bleeding ....................................... 68
Venezuelan encephalitis ............................. 42
venomous bites ......................... 142, 146, 179
VetWrap ............................. 29, 30, 33, 163
vomiting .................................................. 127
WEE .................................................. 41, 42, 64
West Nile ......................................... 41, 42, 64
West Nile Viral Encephalitis ...................... 42
Western Equine Encephalitis ............... 42, 64
Zimecterin ................................................. 59

# About the Author

**Dr. Christian O'Malley** graduated from NC State College of Veterinary Medicine in 1996. Since graduation, Dr. O'Malley has devoted his practice exclusively to equines. A large part of Dr. O'Malley's practice is ambulatory, so he is well rehearsed in all aspects of caring for the ailing equine in the field setting.

Dr. O'Malley and his wife Dr. Amy are the owners of Warrenton Animal Clinic, a mixed animal practice they started in 1999. Dealing with equine emergencies is a common occurrence for Dr. Chris since he is the only equine veterinarian available in the surrounding horse country.

In 2005, Dr. O'Malley began to compile his experience and knowledge of equine emergencies into his book entitled "*Horse 911: Dr. O'Malley's Veterinary Emergency Handbook*". This handbook is packed with concise, easy to understand information pertaining to equine emergencies. The sole purpose of the book is to provide the horse owner an opportunity to help themselves and their horse in a time of crisis. Dr. O'Malley feels that horse owners in particular are more attuned to the health and care of their horses as compared to other pet owners. For this reason, he wants all horse owners to be knowledgeable in the well-being of their horse.

On a personal note, Dr. O'Malley is an avid outdoorsman and enjoys hunting, fishing and camping. When he's not working he stays busy with his wife raising their three children.

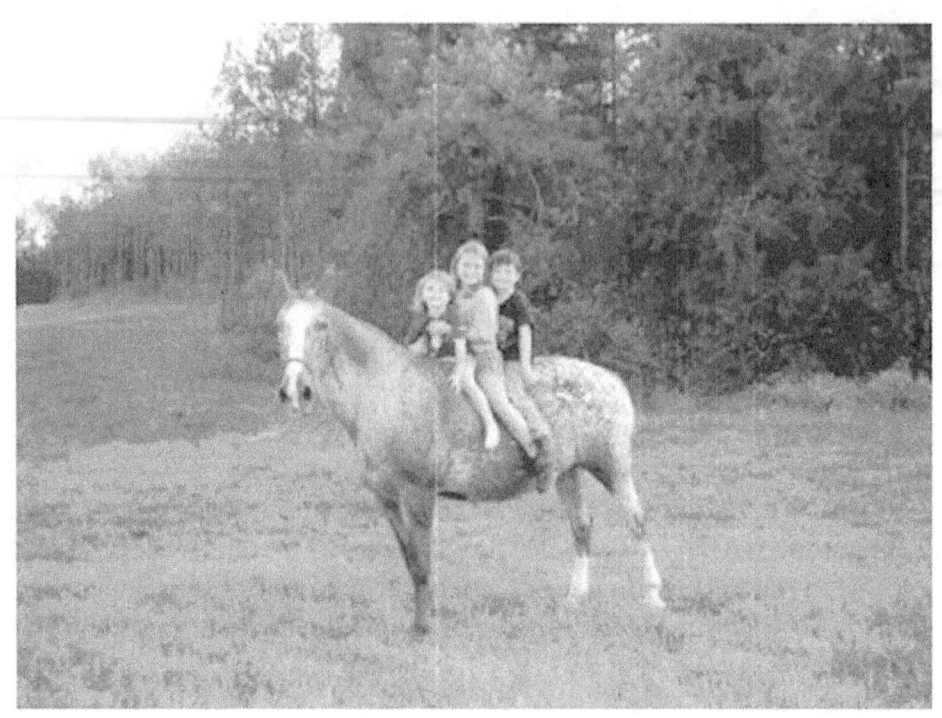

www.ingramcontent.com/pod-product-compliance
Lightning Source LLC
Chambersburg PA
CBHW082114230426
43671CB00015B/2701